Praise for *8 Ways to Hope*

"The reader will finish this wonderful book with a deeper understanding of hope and how to cultivate it. Thank you, Dr. Miller, for sending this gift out into the world."
—Michael McGee, MD, DLFAPA, author of *The Joy of Recovery*

"Hope is a superpower—it helps people solve problems, recover from injuries, and have better relationships. Rich with storytelling, this book is full of optimism and purpose. It shows how to use hope to lead a more fulfilling life."
—Scott T. Walters, PhD,
Regents Professor, School of Public Health,
University of North Texas Health Science Center

"A profoundly satisfying, enlightening book."
—Monty Roberts, author of *The Man Who Listens to Horses*

"Combine great passion for science with deep reverence for the transcendent. Mix in attention to detail and add a large dollop of artistic sensibility. The result is this exquisite gem, which helps us better understand and find multiple paths to hope. In his trademark style, Dr. Miller takes complex science and presents it in language that anyone can understand and use. You may not know it yet, but you need this book—we all do."
—David B. Rosengren, PhD,
President and CEO, Prevention Research Institute

"At a time when it feels like hope belongs on the 'most endangered' list, this book shows hope is still very much alive. I found myself laughing at times and even tearing up over Dr. Miller's stories of everyday heroes who live with and spread hope."
—Annam Manthiram, nonprofit executive, Dallas

"Dr. Miller uses science, history, the arts, and a lifetime of personal experience to illuminate each facet of hope. He reveals ways to see, grasp, hold onto, and live in hope."
—Charles H. Bombardier, PhD,
Department of Rehabilitation Medicine,
University of Washington

8 WAYS TO HOPE

Also Available

8 WAYS TO
HOPE

CHARTING A PATH
THROUGH UNCERTAIN TIMES

William R. Miller, PhD

THE GUILFORD PRESS
New York   London

Copyright © 2024 The Guilford Press
A Division of Guilford Publications, Inc.
370 Seventh Avenue, Suite 1200, New York, NY 10001
www.guilford.com

Printed in the United States of America

Last digit is print number: 9   8   7   6   5   4   3   2   1

Library of Congress Cataloging-in-Publication Data
Names: Miller, William R. (William Richard), author.
Title: 8 ways to hope: charting a path through uncertain times / William
    R. Miller.
Other titles: Eight ways to hope
Description: New York: The Guilford Press, [2024] | Includes
    bibliographical references and index. |
Identifiers: LCCN 2024012017 | ISBN 9781462551286 (paperback) |
    ISBN 9781462554928 (cloth)
Subjects: LCSH: Hope. | Uncertainty. | BISAC: PSYCHOLOGY /
    Mental Health | SOCIAL SCIENCE / Social Work
Classification: LCC BF575.H56 M55 2024 | DDC
    152.4—dc23/eng/20240603
LC record available at *https://lccn.loc.gov/2024012017*

to Dr. Carolina Yahne
who lives hope

Contents

Preface

Our society was reeling from the COVID-19 pandemic, economic woes, global warming, political polarization, wars and rumors of wars, and the endless onslaught of tragedy on broadcast news. I was talking with my editor at The Guilford Press about the need for hope, and I began considering how I might approach a new book on the subject. I have enjoyed learning and writing about universal human experiences such as ambivalence, empathy, faith, and love. But what about hope?

My usual strategy when exploring a broad topic like this has been to immerse myself in published research to find out what has been learned not just in my own field of psychology, but also in related human sciences and professions, to discover what might be relevant and of interest to most people. What quickly became evident to me is that hope is not a monolithic phenomenon but rather a rich array of interrelated human experiences. Together they are like a precious diamond reflecting how we view the future, and it is when the diamond is turned that its different facets shine. I was smitten.

What I hope to do for you is to rotate this fascinating gem that has been with us at least as long as written language, considering one aspect at a time. I am bolstered by butterflies that, to my delight, regularly sail past my office window, having decided that the patio outside is their playground. They don't live for long, just a couple of months from eggs to splendid adults with bright yellow and black tiger-striped wings. They celebrate airborne mating dances to fulfill hope for the next generation and the coming year. But I stray.

Some facets of hope will catch your eye more directly than others. Where each of us grounds our hope will vary. Some rest it on statistical probabilities; others see possibilities. Some live with the heartache of desire for what should be or simply trust that it shall be. Some rest their hope on a bedrock of meaning, while others keep on moving, persisting toward the horizon they envision. There are high-hope optimists, and long-shot gamblers, and those who hope against hope. We are on this lifelong journey together, toting our hope-filled backpacks of varied sizes and colors. Let's unpack them.

CHAPTER 1

Finding Our Way in the Dark

Hope is being able to see that there is light
despite all of the darkness.
— DESMOND TUTU

Those who do not hope for the unexpected
will not find it.
— HERACLITUS

Of all the unique wedding gifts that the couple had received, it was certainly the strangest: a large clay jar with a sealed lid, accompanied by a stern warning never to open it. Of course, curiosity prevailed. As soon as the jar was opened, out flew a swarm of plagues. They clapped the cap back onto the jar, but it was too late; the afflictions had been loosed on the world.

In conveying this ancient story from mythology, a translator in 1508 mistakenly rendered the Greek work for a jar—*pithos*—as "box," and five centuries later it continues to be known as Pandora's box. A New Mexico governor once garbled it further by exclaiming, "Well, that opens up a whole box of Pandoras!" Perhaps he thought they were cigars. An important detail that is often omitted in telling this classic story is the single thing that remained in the jar after all the grim afflictions had escaped. It was hope.

Hope is always about the unknown, particularly the future. We might *wish* for a different past, but would not *hope* for it. We also don't hope for that which seems certain to occur or has already happened. Actually there is an exception here, because we can be hopeful about the past until we learn what actually transpired. "I hope you slept well." "I hope our team won yesterday." Marooned on a desert island, we might wistfully imagine what is happening in the world during our absence. Even here, though, hope pertains to what we will learn in the future about what has already occurred. In an era of near-instantaneous information and communication, the period of hoping prior to knowing has been greatly diminished.

Hope is anticipated possibility, something that we do when confronting uncertainty. In saying "do," I mean not merely overt actions. Although hope can take the form of observable behavior, what we do when faced with uncertainty also includes aspects of the inner world such as choosing, attending, thinking, feeling, and remembering, all of which can be done hopefully. Hope is all about anticipation of what is not yet. It is a liminal space, a threshold to what may yet be. Indeed, hope can critique and transform the present.[1]

There seems to be an inherent human desire to hope, especially during dark times.[2] Like night vision, hope is a way of seeing in the dark, although it may take a while for your vision to adjust. Through many threats and dangers, Dr. Martin Luther King Jr. held on to his dream for the future: "We must accept finite disappointment, but never lose infinite hope." It is the stuff of visions that sustain us and of songs proclaiming that we *shall* overcome.

The essence of hope is envisioned betterment, and it serves us well. It comes hardwired in human nature to dream a better future,

> With what is happening in your life now and in the world around you, what are your three fondest hopes?

helping us to carry on and survive. Hope "springs eternal in the human breast,"[3] especially in times like the present plagued by war, a pandemic, global warming, social polarization, and crushing economic disparity.[4] It arises in the midst of obstacles and uncertainty, when the present is troubled and the future is unclear. It is a universal human experience that lives in the realm of not-yet, searching beyond how things *are* to envision what *could* be. Animals respond to the present and remember the past, but so far as we know, contemplating possible distant futures is a uniquely human experience. People and many mammals grieve after losing a companion, but *anticipatory* grief about a coming loss requires an imagined future. We can envision what *might* be, and that is where hope lives.

Varieties of Hope

Hope is an experience that everyone knows, yet exactly what *is* it? Although it's familiar, hope can also be fleeting, like the tiger swallowtail and the hummingbird that are winging outside my window as I write this. It has an elusive, intangible quality that can be difficult to pin down in a definition. As we shall see, this is in part because, like butterflies and birds, hope comes in varied forms. As I read background research for this book, it quickly became clear to me that hope is not just one single thing. It is complex, with many faces, forms, and foundations that are complementary aspects of the same experience.[5] Hope can be a feeling, thought, action, vision, a life force, and a way of seeing or being. It stands amid the abiding spiritual triad of faith, hope, and love.[6] Two definitions dating from the 11th century portrayed hope as a stepping-stone up to a higher level and as an oasis in the midst of a wasteland.[7] It is all of these things, no one of which captures its full essence. A diamond therefore seems an apt metaphor for hope. It has many facets, great beauty, and is among the hardest and most precious of gems. A diamond may be given as a sign of hope and commitment.

There can be a downside to hope. One of the most famous gemstones is the large blue Hope Diamond, so named for one of its many owners, some of whom, ironically, met with misfortune and tragedy, giving rise to the stone's alleged curse.[8] The Greek myth of Pandora could suggest that the hope left behind in the jar was merely another curse.[9] Hope has many different aspects. When speaking about hope, people may be describing just one narrow part of it. For example, hope might be equated with an unwarranted optimism that, while comforting, could undermine the perceived urgency of action. Living in a dreamworld of hope, one may miss the joy of the present.

Yet the usual results of hope are overwhelmingly positive, as we see in the chapters ahead that consider many aspects of hope, turning the diamond to explore its facets in how we may respond when faced with uncertainty. There is more than one way of hoping. Before the final chapter we will have considered eight different facets of hope, varied ways of seeing beyond the present to the not-yet.

Hope and Fear

Besides hope, there is another universal human experience that also dwells in the land of not-yet, imagining what might be. It is fear. In the human mind, both hope and fear project images of what could come to pass, and both can be powerfully motivating. They are alternative lenses through which to view an uncertain future, and to some extent they counteract each other, although they can also coexist.[10] I am hopeful for the next generations, including my own children's and grandchildren's futures, and I also fret for what life may bring them. Hope and fear have a contentious relationship, and we each choose how to make peace with them. Hope tends to expand our horizons, while fear contracts them.

No matter the year, the world affords ample evidence to justify despair, and we are understandably wired by our evolutionary history to pay special attention to any negative information.[11] Fear is our built-in smoke alarm for survival. If something is even remotely a potential threat, we want to know about it. Obligingly, there are news media and websites offering a constant diet of danger and darkness. When there is insufficient local calamity for today's news, there are always distressing tragedies to report from elsewhere. As when passing a traffic accident, a part of us just feels compelled to look: poverty, violence, disease and death, natural disasters, global warming, and human inhumanity.

Yet fear is not the only voice we can hear, and it does not deserve the last word. In the midst of travail, hope remains as an antidote to fear. Whenever biblical angels speak, their first words are usually a comforting message of hope: "Fear not." Hope and fear suppress

What are your significant fears now, and do you have related hopes?

each other. As a very old hardwired survival response, fear is quick and often is the first experience. What happens next, however, is a matter of choice. Fear can predominate, leading to fight, flight, or just shutting down. Hope opens up different paths. Amid the Great Depression in 1933, President Franklin Roosevelt famously declared that "we have nothing to fear but fear itself."[12] Fear can shut down the creative capacity to find better ways and even the will to find them. Hope is about finding both the will and a way forward.[13]

It is quite possible, as mentioned, to experience both hope and fear together. They may urge us in opposite directions, but we still get to choose which path to follow. The dread of dark potential can fuel an urgent quest for a brighter future. Courage is not the absence of fear, but moving ahead with hope in spite of it. Exploring the varieties of hope is an alternative to sinking into the immobilizing mire of hopelessness and fear. It can also be useful to walk with others who have walked the same path through darkness and emerged on the other side.

Hopelessness

In Dante Alighieri's 14th-century *Divine Comedy* an inscription stands above the gates to hell: *Abandon all hope, you who enter here.* Despair, the total loss of hope, can be hellish indeed. Hopelessness can follow from persistent adversity, significant losses, or trauma. It is a classic component of clinical depression and contributes to risk for suicide.[14] In the course of life I have experienced periods of significant depression myself, and a striking aspect of it for me was the vanishing of my characteristic optimism. It was one of the earliest changes that I noticed before I realized what was happening. I had written about major depression and had treated people who were suffering with it but had never experienced it firsthand. Happily, depression is normally quite treatable, and over a period of months my positive outlook on life returned.

It is normal to grant yourself the benefit of the doubt, viewing yourself more generously than others might. It is a common human tendency to take credit for what goes well and to attribute negative outcomes to bad luck, adverse circumstances, or other people. By contrast, depressed people do just the opposite. They often blame themselves for all kinds of adversity while being dismissive about taking credit for what is good. Their views of their own abilities and the controllability of life tend to be dimmer, though sometimes more accurate than the norm—a phenomenon known as *depressive realism*.[15] Isn't that depressing?

There is good reason, however, to think positively about yourself and others because, as discussed in later chapters, that which you expect is more likely to come true. When you start to fear something, you begin looking for it and then you start finding it. Hopelessness fosters helplessness—to give up rather than "to take arms against a sea of troubles, and by opposing end them."[16] Fear combined with low hope encourages passivity and avoidance rather than active coping, which in turn becomes a self-fulfilling prophecy. Your level of hope, whether high or low, is thus mirrored in what you do and becomes a way of life.

The Science of Hope

How much do we know about hope? I was fascinated to find out. In 1959, the eminent psychiatrist Karl Menninger accurately bemoaned the scarcity of research on this "basic but elusive ingredient" in healing: "When it comes to hope, our shelves are bare. The journals are silent."[17] He was right, but it's no longer true. Just half a century later in Menninger's own discipline alone there were 49 definitions and 32 measurement instruments for hope.[18] With the burgeoning of behavioral science over the same period, research and scholarship on hope are now abundant in ecology,[19] economics,[20]

medicine,[21] nursing,[22] philosophy,[23] political science,[24] psychology,[25] sociology,[26] and theology.[27] Clearly there is broad interest in
understanding this universal human experience. Part of what this
book offers is a distillation of hundreds of articles and books published over the decades since Menninger lamented their absence.
For readers interested in the details of particular ideas or findings,
documentation is provided in endnotes to each chapter. If what
engages you is the overall story, just read on.

People Who Hope

Hope can be measured; in fact, many instruments are available.
This makes it possible to learn how hope is related to other aspects
of health and personality. People who hope stand out from others
in a wide variety of ways. Within a large volume of research on the
subject, those who are high in hope have been found to also:

- Be better at solving problems[28]
- Experience a higher quality of life even in the face of adver-
  sity[29]
- Be more resilient and persistent[30]
- Transcend the difficult present, finding greater meaning
  and purpose in life[31]
- Be more engaged and satisfied with their work, and be bet-
  ter at it[32]
- Have higher creativity, adaptivity, and academic achieve-
  ment[33]
- Recover more readily after a disabling injury[34]
- Experience better outcomes in counseling and psychother-
  apy[35]

Hope can be quite specific. You might hope *for* something in particular to happen. Research shows that *self-efficacy*—the belief in your ability to accomplish a specific task—predicts success in actually doing it.[36] Yet hope is so much larger than wishing for specific things. It can also be a far broader perspective, a positive orientation toward and investment in the future.[37] For example, with a lifetime of observation and reflection, the French scientist–philosopher and theologian Pierre Teilhard de Chardin concluded that history and humankind are systematically evolving toward a profoundly positive "omega point."[38] There are setbacks and switchbacks along the way, but ultimately there is a progressive maturation. Shortly before his death, Martin Luther King Jr. proclaimed a similarly hopeful message that "the arc of the moral universe is long but it bends toward justice."[39] Such big-picture perspectives of a bright far horizon help people transcend and endure dark times, like the light at the far end of a long tunnel. Hope is a vital component of what is known as our *psychological capital*—the development of perseverance and adaptiveness to succeed at challenging tasks.[40] It is vital when coping with serious and prolonged stress.[41]

Not just a characteristic of individuals, hope is communicable to and sharable with others. It can become a *collective* orientation within families and groups, and even as part of a society's common vision of the future.[42] Both hope and fear are choral and contagious and thereby are motivational themes found in political discourse that can sway decision making. Like common colds, we give them to each other.

Given the plethora of positive characteristics with which it is associated, hope might be considered a master virtue. It is a positive orientation of mind and heart toward your own future or that of the world at large. Hope is a chosen perspective, an alternative to fear and despair. We're not required to hope, but if we decide to do so there are at least eight ways from which to choose. Let's begin.

TAKING IT PERSONALLY: HOPE

- Have you ever gone through a time when hope felt particularly important to you? Are you struggling with a personal experience or global event now where hope might help you in the same way?

- On a scale of 1–10, how hopeful are you compared to other people?

- Looking to the future, what are two or three things you really hope for?

CHAPTER 2

Desire

The natural flights of the human mind are not from pleasure to pleasure but from hope to hope.
—SAMUEL JOHNSON

Any time someone tells me that I can't do something, I want to do it more.
—TAYLOR SWIFT

Her mother died when she was only 2, and at age 4 she contracted tuberculosis that curved her spine and caused her to walk with a limp, making her unable to run and play like other girls. She became a prolific reader, and inspired by the novels of Charles Dickens, Jane Addams developed a passion to alleviate the suffering of the poor. She longed to make a useful contribution in the world, a desire that propelled her through a long life and legacy of accomplishments. With her friend Ellen Starr she cofounded and resided in Hull House, the first U.S. settlement house for living among and serving the poor and immigrants of Chicago. She rose to prominence in national and international women's organizations. Addams encouraged women's "ambition and aspirations" long before women won the right to vote, and she is recognized as a founding mother of social work as a new profession for women. She was the first woman to receive an

honorary degree from Yale University and the second to
be awarded the Nobel Peace Prize.[1]

What do you hope for? Perhaps the most common use of
the word *hope* is to describe something that you wish for, want, or
desire. Every language on the face of the earth has a way of saying "I
want."[2] Infants learn how to communicate their desires long before
they develop spoken language. In musical theater there is usually
an "I want" song in the first act, in which protagonists express
their desires, hopes, dreams. Some classics are "Somewhere over the
Rainbow" in *The Wizard of Oz,* "The Music of the Night" in *Phan-
tom of the Opera,* and "My Shot" in *Hamilton.*

The beginning of hope is to want. Desire is an *essential* aspect
of hoping. You can estimate probability (Chapter 3) and envision
possibility (Chapter 4), but it's not hope unless and until you also
want it. Energy enters through this facet of desire and lights up the
diamond of hope.

Sometimes what we call *hope* is pure wishing. It's what I experience when after traveling for 2 weeks, having eaten too well and
exercised too little, I am about to step on the bathroom scale at
home, hoping for a temporary exemption from the laws of nature.
That might even be called hope against hope, but I have reserved
that term for a deeper discussion in Chapter 9.

The power of hopeful desire is encoded in the Greek myth of
Pygmalion, a king of Cyprus and a gifted sculptor, who fashioned
an ivory statue of a perfect woman whom he named Galatea. The
statue was so beautiful that he wound up falling in love with her.
He would kiss and caress her; he laid gifts at her feet and built an
elaborate bed for her on which she could rest. On the day of the
festival of the goddess Aphrodite, Pygmalion went to the temple to

offer a sacrificial gift, longing for a wife who would be as lovely as his sculpture. On returning home, a surprise awaited him. When he kissed Galatea on the mouth as usual, he thought that he had sensed the warmth of breath. He kissed her again, and indeed her lips were soft and warm. Aphrodite, whom the Romans called Venus, had brought Galatea to life in fulfillment of his hope and prayer, as in the 19th-century Italian story of Pinocchio.

Hopes are not always fulfilled of course but desire can contribute to reality. The mythical king's name was bestowed on the *Pygmalion effect* in psychology, a short summary of which is that "what you get is what you see," for better or worse. As is discussed in Chapter 4, seeing possibility in others can call it forth. In the popular musical *My Fair Lady* and George Bernard Shaw's play *Pygmalion* on which it was based, a phonetics professor envisions how an impoverished flower girl could be transformed into a sophisticated lady by changing how she speaks, and he desires it to happen if only to win a bet. Such self-fulfilling prophecies of expectation have been shown to occur in education,[3] in leadership and management,[4] and in military and workplace settings.[5]

Desire is necessary but not sufficient for hoping. To have hope, at least these three conditions are necessary: First, you must have a goal or purpose in mind, some uncertain future occurrence that is the object of your hope. Without an aspiration, you have nothing for which to hope. Second, you must desire it. And third, what you hope for must seem possible (Chapter 4) even if improbable (Chapter 3). You might wish that you could talk to Nelson Mandela or Cleopatra, but you would not hope to do so.[6] Desire without possibility is not hope.[7] You also don't usually hope that the sun will rise tomorrow, because it's so sure to happen.[8] Hope is for that which lies somewhere between certain and impossible.[9] It doesn't have to be *very* possible. In fact, what you desire may seem close to impossible, but you can still hope for it. Commercial and political advertising can suggest all three key components of hope: an ideal goal, reasons to desire it, and an ostensible way to achieve it.[10]

The potency of wanting can vary. It might be a fairly superficial hope, like a taste preference: "I hope they have spumoni ice cream today." As importance increases, so does desire: "I really hope we win this game today" or "I hope I get this job." Depth of desire can even be profound, like a desert wanderer's thirsty need to find water or an urgent longing for relief from intense suffering.

In developing the method of motivational interviewing for helping people change and grow, Steve Rollnick and I distinguished between two motivational components: importance and confidence.[11] As with hope, motivation for change requires just enough of both elements. Our work began with trying to help people change their harmful use of alcohol.[12] Often the obstacle we encountered with drinkers was that they didn't believe it was *important* enough to change. "I feel fine. I don't drink any more than my friends do, and it's not a problem for me. I *could* quit if I wanted to, but why would I do that?" They didn't see a persuasive *why* to change what they were doing, a sufficient reason to *want* to change. Other clients had a *why* and a desire to change but couldn't see a *how*. They knew well enough that change was important for them, but they had little confidence that it could happen. "I've tried and tried to quit, but I always wind up going right back to smoking. It's too hard; I just can't do it." Some people lacked both importance and confidence, having neither the will nor a way to change. The ones who rarely came in for help were those who had both the *why* and the *how* of change, because they were already busy doing it.

Hope is like that too. One of the most widely regarded theories is that of psychologist Charles Snyder, who devoted much of his career to studying hope.[13] He taught that there are two vital components of hope—will and way. By "will" he meant a sense of personal agency, being generally able to accomplish your goals. Snyder's "way" element is finding one or more potentially effective paths to try in pursuing a goal. He observed that the saying "Where there's a will, there's a way" isn't quite accurate.[14] There are people who wish for change and clearly regard it to be important, yet see no way to accomplish it. Will without way might be called despair. Those who are caught up in protracted conflict may yearn for peace yet have little or no belief that it can ever be realized.[15] They have given up, and the conflict continues. From Snyder's perspective of needing both will and way, they lack hope. You need both desire and possibility.

> What in your life have you *desired* but didn't regard to be *possible*? How did you respond to or resolve that situation?

By the way, hope does not have to rely on confidence in your own ability. You may believe that positive change will be possible through others' efforts without requiring your own active participation.[16] This is a somewhat lazy kind of hoping because, like cynicism, it requires nothing of you. Such assurance might be based on faith in human nature, a charismatic leader, free-market forces, God, the slow-bending arc of the moral universe toward justice, or the ultimate power of love. At the heart of such an optimistic external-source-of-hope view, things will all work out well in the end without your having to do much to help it happen.

It's also possible to have confidence in such external forces and want to do your own part as well. Large changes are often the cumulative result of countless small individual efforts. The demoralizing thought "What difference could I possibly make?" overlooks this snowballing contribution of many personal choices, as through small financial contributions, voting, recycling, or random acts of kindness. The sustaining hopeful vision here is of cooperating with and joining in the momentum of larger forces at work. It is living as if the possibility you hope for is already on the way. "Be the change you want to see in the world" is a distillation of a longer teaching from Mahatma Gandhi that ends with "We need not wait to see what others do." Michael Jackson captured the same spirit in his song "The Man in the Mirror," emphasizing that making the world a better place begins with changing yourself.

Hopeful people are more likely to try to reach their goals. In physical rehabilitation, for example, patients with higher levels of hope regain more function and ability to take care of themselves.[17] It doesn't have to be a general optimism, which I consider in Chapter 5. Confidence in your specific ability to accomplish a particular task predicts actually completing it,[18] and so does a stated intention to do it.[19] Your own hope affects what you will do.

Hope for Others

In addition to what you want for yourself, you also experience hope for others. In everyday conversation people express such desire for someone's well-being and happiness:

I hope you have a great trip.

May you sleep well tonight.

Bon appétit!

Safe travels!

Feel better soon!

Saying "Break a leg" to a performer who's about to go on stage is a supportive wish for their success, a kind of reverse incantation rather than saying "good luck," which might be superstitiously regarded as bad luck. "I hope . . ." statements can wish good for people for their own sake, like unconditional support and affection.[20]

Notice that expressing hope for others can imply passivity. The hoper may not be doing anything to make the wish more likely to be fulfilled and may believe there's nothing they can do. "I hope" is not in itself an offer of help except perhaps in the form of prayer: "I hope and pray" or "I pray that you. . . ." It's an inexpensive kind of hoping. Thoughts and prayers that are offered on someone's behalf may be equally fleeting.

Benevolent hopes can be voiced for many reasons. They might be self-serving hopes, expressed with some anticipation of personal favor or gain in return, or they can convey genuine sympathy and a desire for the other's well-being. Sympathy is feeling *for*, imagining what a person in their situation must be experiencing. Effective acting in theater or film can offer a glimpse inside another's emotion and may evoke sympathetic tears. Howard Thurman observed that "I can sympathize only when I see myself in another's place."[21] Still, sympathy is more a matter of envisioning than of actually experiencing another's pain. A deeper understanding is empathy—feeling *with* rather than *for* someone. There is a personal connection of shared experience rather than just mentally imagining what it must be like. Although empathic responding can be measured reliably by observers,[22] the *experience* of empathy occurs in a relationship, in live person-to-person interaction.

In any event, it does matter what you hope for others, and such hope involves not only desire, but also expectation for their well-being. The previously mentioned Pygmalion effect can occur

in medical and behavioral health care. The outcome of an illness
or psychological crisis is shaped not only by the person's own hope,
but also by the hope of their caregivers.[23] The staff of three resi-
dential alcoholism treatment programs were informed that, based
on psychological testing, some of their patients had high alcoholism recovery potential (HARP) and were likely to show remarkable
improvement with treatment.[24] When the staff rated each patient
at discharge, they reported that the HARP patients had indeed
been significantly more motivated, punctual, cooperative, and better looking, and as trying harder in recovery and having better prog-
noses, a prediction that turned out to be true. During the year following treatment, the HARP patients had fewer drinking episodes
and longer spans of abstinence and were more likely to be employed.
However, the researchers had a secret. Unbeknown to the staff, the
patients who were identified as HARP had actually been chosen
at random and not on the basis of psychological testing. The only
difference was that the staff were given to expect that the HARP
patients had an unusually high potential for good recovery.

Expectations about others can also be detrimental. People
in close intimate relationships have hopes and fears about their
romantic partners. For various reasons, some people are particularly sensitive to and concerned about being jilted. Such rejection-
sensitive people are more likely to have breakups in their romantic
relationships. What may account for this? A study of young couples
who had been dating for just a few months included a 20-minute
videotaped discussion of a relationship issue on which there had
been disagreement. The topics included commitment, sex, other
friendships, and time together. Each partner's verbal and nonverbal responses were classified via a complex observation system.
Negative behaviors during these discussions included complaints,

putdowns, denials of responsibility, negative voice tone and facial expressions, as well as adverse "mind-reading" interpretations of the partner's motivations or mindset. For women but not for men, those with high sensitivity to rejection expressed many more negative responses during the conflict conversation, and their partners reported feeling angrier with them afterward.[25] In other words, fear of rejection can breed anticipatory negativity, which in turn invites actual rejection. Why did sensitivity to rejection predict negative behavior only for women? It's unclear, but the authors speculated that conflict in relationships may have different meaning and importance for women than for men.

Hopes are not always benevolent, even toward oneself. The oath "cross my heart and hope to die," which was first recorded in 1908, invokes a wicked consequence for dishonesty. Expressed hopes can reflect ill will. Depending on tone of voice and nonverbal cues, seeming words of hope can convey sarcasm (I hope you enjoy your ill-gotten gain) or even threat (I hope you lock your doors at night). Hopes can directly convey malice, a desire for harm to come to someone (To the person who stole my case of energy drinks: I hope you can't sleep at night). To wish for the victory of one's own team or military is to hope for the defeat or destruction of another.[26] Do such malign desires, like a hex or curse, actually influence outcomes?

In a classic 1942 journal article, the physiologist Walter Cannon (who coined the term *fight or flight response*) documented wide-ranging reports of inexplicable sudden deaths in various primitive cultures soon after the victim had violated a taboo or been cursed by a medicine man or an enemy.[27] The victims quickly fell ill and became weak although no medical cause could be identified. Treatments were to no avail, and they died within a day or so of being cursed. Some simply accepted that their death was inevitable and succumbed. It overrode or supplanted their desire to live. For these mysterious "voodoo" deaths Cannon proposed a biological explanation that has held up rather well through subsequent neuroscience discoveries of hormones and brain chemicals related to fear that can trigger cardiac arrhythmia and vascular collapse.[28]

Self-Fulfilling Prophecies

The term *self-fulfilling prophecy* was coined in 1948 by Robert Merton, an American sociologist who said that people "respond not only to the objective facts and features of a situation, but also, and at times primarily, to the meaning this situation has for them. And once they have assigned some meaning to the situation, their subsequent behavior and some of the consequences of that behavior are determined by the ascribed meaning."[29] In other words, what they do helps it come true. This happens in three steps. First, based on superficial characteristics, people develop false perceptions of others that include expectations of how they will behave. Professionals with influence (such as physicians, nurses, teachers, and coaches) likewise develop such perceptions and expectations about those under their care. Second, whether consciously or not, the perceiver treats people differently based on these expectations. Finally, people react in ways that confirm the perceiver's initial beliefs.[30] The perceivers are often blithely unaware of how their own actions affect others' behavior to confirm their beliefs.[31] For example, suspecting that someone (or many people) will harbor ill will toward him, a man tests his assumption by insulting or provoking them and, sure enough, they respond with hostility. In this way expectations, like a virus, can replicate themselves in an individual or group, often without awareness, and mightily resist efforts to remove them.[32]

Beyond any actual change in the other's behavior, expectations can also bias your *interpretation* of actions in a way that confirms your expectations even in the absence of any real evidence. For example, what would happen if normal people who had never received a mental diagnosis or suffered pathological symptoms were admitted to a psychiatric hospital as patients? Would they be discovered to be sane? In a classic study,[33] eight such normal men and women presented themselves for evaluation at 12 psychiatric hospitals in five different U.S. states, using a false name and occupation. They complained of hearing voices that spoke the words *empty, hollow,* or *thud.* Otherwise they recounted their actual life history and experiences. All were readily admitted, after which they immediately stopped feigning any symptoms of abnormality and behaved as they normally would. They conversed with patients, publicly kept notes of their experiences, and if asked by the staff how they were feeling they said they felt fine and were not hearing voices. Ordinary behaviors were interpreted by the staff as pathological. For example, lining up early for a meal was interpreted as illustrating the "oral-acquisitive" nature of schizophrenia. Walking in the hallway was interpreted as anxiety. Note taking itself was regarded as paranoid. After various lengths of time behaving normally, all were discharged as "schizophrenic, in remission."

Are there modern parallels to voodoo deaths where negative predictions yield dire outcomes? The pronouncement of a medical prognosis is one possibility of a self-fulfilling prophecy. Just as the announcement of a good (although fictitious) prognosis for the

HARP patients portended their recovery, being told that there is little or no hope may prompt passive acceptance even if the presumption is false. When patients suffer a hemorrhagic stroke, for example, families and health care providers can face a decision of whether to withdraw life-sustaining medical support. The perception of poor prognosis and futility of care can guide a decision to withdraw life support, and a resulting death confirms the prognosis.[34] Yet some people who suffer devastating strokes do survive and recover function. Here is a situation where statistical probabilities based on experience (Chapter 3), as well as the desires and expectations of those involved, can contribute to outcomes.

A dark side of the Pygmalion effect then is that malign predictions of someone's future can also become self-confirming. As an adolescent, Malcolm X had a life-shaping conversation with a high school teacher regarding his career options. Voicing an interest in becoming a lawyer, he was told that this was not a realistic possibility for a Black man. "The more I thought afterwards about what he said, the more uneasy it made me. It just kept treading around in my mind." In contrast, White students with grades lower than Malcolm's were encouraged by the same teacher to pursue their dreams. "It was then that I began to change—inside. I drew away from white people. I came to class, and I [only] answered when called upon. . . . Nobody, including the teachers, could decide what had come over me."[35] He gave up his desire to become an attorney and drifted into a life of robbery and burglary that he would later call "evil." When arrested at age 20, he was sentenced to 10 years in prison, where he earned the nickname "Satan." There are countless such stories in which someone's identity can suddenly shift to and crystallize on the dark side.[36]

Self-confirming expectations also occur at a social level. A false rumor that a bank is about to fail creates a demand for withdrawals that can make the previously false belief come true.[37] Predictions of a product shortage (such as toilet paper) trigger panic buying that empties the store shelves. It can work in both directions. Consumer confidence stimulates spending, confirming perceptions of a strong economy.

What You Want Is What You See

As discussed thus far in this chapter, what you hope for can influence what actually happens. Beyond this, what you desire also influences what you will see and not see. Every day you encounter many kinds of information that you can attend to or ignore, remember or forget, and interpret as you please. People with autism or traumatic brain injury may have difficulty filtering out overstimulation, but normally your brain screens out potentially irrelevant information, allowing you to focus better on what matters.

Some of this brain filtering of input from the eyes, ears, and other sensory organs is hardwired and automatic. Part of it, however, is motivated selection, wishful perceiving if you will. Your hopes and fears also filter what you see—what you will notice and remember and also how you interpret what you experience. Some of this selection process is conscious. We can be at least partially aware of a confirmation bias in choosing to pay more attention to certain news sources, books, and other people who confirm what we already believe and to avoid information that contradicts our current opinions. Beyond such deliberate filtering of information, it is also well documented that confirmation bias can operate without our awareness.[38]

A famous example of blindness through selective attention is a 75-second video that was made for a study at Harvard University and then went viral on the Internet.[39] On the video are two teams with three players each, one wearing white shirts and the other black shirts. Both teams have a basketball that they pass to each other, either through the air or on the bounce. The two teams simultaneously dribble and pass their basketballs while weaving around each other, and the observer's task is to pay attention and count how many times the players in white shirts pass the ball to each other. (In a more difficult version, they try to count aerial and bounce passes separately.) After reporting their counts, the observers in the study were asked whether they had noticed anything unusual in the video. The unexpected 5-second event is a woman wearing a full gorilla suit who casually walks in among the players, turns to face the camera, beats her chest, and then strolls off camera while the ball passing continues around her. Fifty-six percent of those watching the video never noticed the gorilla; even fewer noticed when concentrating on the harder task of counting aerial versus bounce passes. What we're looking for is what we tend to see.

How does the brain decide what to focus on and what to ignore? Two very old and strong motivational brain systems signal you to approach or to avoid what you see.[40] The former might be called a hope system, to seek and approach what you believe to be good. Think of the familiar image of two people running toward each other, eager to be reunited. The other protective system drives you to avoid and run

Are you someone more inclined to move toward hoped-for pleasure or to avoid possible risk and harm?

away from what is bad and dangerous. These systems have obvious survival value—to find nutritious food and avoid predators. Individuals can be predisposed to be much more driven by one of these systems than by the other. Some people are more inclined to seek reward and pleasure, perhaps without giving due attention to attendant risks. Others are high in harm-avoiding motivation and tend to be worriers, anxious about bad things happening to them, more cautious and inhibited. Avoidant motivation may be the understandable result of traumatic experience.

Avoidance seems particularly prone to biasing perception. People high in avoidance motivation tend to be hypervigilant for possible danger, selectively focusing on[41] and remembering negative information.[42] They also tend to interpret neutral or ambiguous information as potentially threatening.[43] Were those raised eyebrows a signal of attraction or of disapproval?

Beyond personality disposition, we more generally see what we want to see. Participants in a taste-testing study were seated at a table with two 8-ounce glasses of beverage in front of them. One glass contained freshly squeezed orange juice and the other a green, nasty-looking, thick and chunky, foul-smelling "veggie smoothy." They were asked to smell both glasses and told that they would be drinking one of them. The computer in front of them would randomly decide which full glass of beverage they were to drink by showing them either a number between 1 and 26 or a letter from the alphabet. A number meant orange juice and a letter meant green goop (or vice versa). The computer then briefly flashed an ambiguous character that could be seen as either a B or a 13. Whichever one meant orange juice, that's what 82 percent of them saw.[44] When faced with ambiguity, we are more likely to see what we hope to see.

Lending Hope

Finally, desire can create hope, and hope encourages us to take action.[45] Directly witnessing suffering is a common motivation to search compassionately for ways to cure or alleviate medical, psychological, and social adversity. My own first exposure to addiction was as a young psychology intern on an inpatient alcoholism treatment ward for military veterans. Knowing almost nothing about this topic, I spent the summer listening to patients (all men at the time) describe how their lives had gradually become entwined with and destroyed by alcohol. It became a primary focus of my career, and at the outset colleagues asked me why I would choose to devote my life to such a grim and hopeless condition. I soon learned that their stereotypes were mistaken, and I now say that I have spent 50 years in addiction treatment and research precisely because the outcomes are so *good*. In fact, the vast majority of people do recover, and you don't need subtle psychological tests to see the difference. The malign and circular prediction is simply false: that you have to let people "hit bottom" and suffer sufficiently before they will be motivated to do anything.[46] We don't do that with cancer, heart disease, depression, or many other recurring conditions where prevention and early treatment are effective. Recognizing the metabolic syndrome of *prediabetes* has fostered early identification and intervention before diabetes can inflict its severe consequences and disability. A call to recognize *preaddiction* holds similar promise to reduce suffering and mortality related to the use of alcohol and other drugs.[47]

When someone lacks hope, you can lend them some of yours—whichever variety of hope you have to offer that might help them.[48] It's not a matter of installing hope so much as evoking it, calling it forth.[49] Hope has long been recognized as a vital ingredient in healing and change, and it's a well-documented characteristic of more effective helpers.[50] People with high hope generally have more goals, set more challenging objectives for themselves, are happier and less distressed, and recover better and faster.[51] Question your assumptions about what someone cannot do.[52] When people seem trapped in hopelessness, share your vision of what is possible as well as your own desire for their happiness and well-being. Hope is a place where you can sit together on the threshold of what can be.

In sum, desire is a good launchpad for hope, a motivation to do something. What outcomes do you want? Choose an objective that you care about and toward which you could take action. What could you do and contribute toward this hope that matters to you?[53] Desire alone won't get it done, but it's a good starting point and an essential component of hope.

TAKING IT PERSONALLY: DESIRE

- Can you think of a time when you were a Pygmalion for someone? When has your own hope or belief in someone helped a dream become reality?

- Who in your own life has served as a Pygmalion for you, seeing potential that you did not see in yourself?

- Think of something that you hope to do. On this 10-point scale, how *important* would you say it is for you to do it?

0	1	2	3	4	5	6	7	8	9	10
Not at all important									Extremely important	

- And how *confident* are you that you will be able to do it if you decide to do it?

0	1	2	3	4	5	6	7	8	9	10
Not at all confident										Completely confident

- Finally, how much do you *want* to do it?

0	1	2	3	4	5	6	7	8	9	10
No desire at all to do it									Strong desire to do it	

- What do these three numbers tell you about your *hope* to do it?

CHAPTER 3

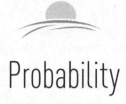

Probability

I always have hope, but I'm a realist.
—JONATHAN CAPEHART[1]

Hope is the feeling you have that the feeling
you have isn't permanent.
—JEAN KERR

When I was diagnosed with early prostate cancer, the oncologist reviewed the various alternatives available to me and asked what I was most comfortable with as a next step. One option was to "watch and wait" to see how the cancer progressed. My natural question was "What does the science have to say about what would be best for me?" I wanted to base my health decision on the best available evidence, and the doctor's answer surprised me: "There's not enough research to say." What? After skin cancers, this is the most common form of cancer in men, and we don't even know what to recommend? I know how to read and conduct clinical trials, so I went to the medical library and found that it was true. At the time I could find only two large controlled trials comparing differ-ent treatments for prostate cancer. The better of the two studies came from Scandinavia, where health outcomes

are well documented, and it showed basically that surgery
was a better choice for men under 65, whereas if you're
over 65 something else is likely to kill you first. I chose
to have surgery, and 14 years later I'm still cancer free. I
don't know whether I'm cured from any recurrence, but
I'm content with how I went about making the decision.
I prefer to consider the available evidence when making
choices. As W. Edwards Deming once quipped: "In God
we trust. All others please bring data."

When the future is in doubt, a reasonable thing to wonder is "How
hopeful should I be?" This question points to another way of thinking about hope, which is probability—the odds that a particular
event is going to take place. Entire occupations focus on estimating
the likelihood that certain things will occur based on known facts.
Bookmakers set odds on the outcome of sporting events like football and horse racing; matchmakers and computer algorithms try
to foretell relationship compatibility. Aptitude tests are designed to
anticipate how well individuals will fare in education or particular
occupations, and pollsters seek to predict the outcome of elections.
Forecasters predict the weather and the stock market, while doctors and actuaries are asked to estimate how long people are going
to live. When poised to hope, something that we naturally want to
know is "What are the chances?"

Actually, people do differ in how much they want to know
when faced with uncertainty. Some of us like to find out as much as
possible before making a decision,
whereas others are content to have sufficient information to make a *good-
enough* choice. These preferences can
apply even with small matters like

> What is your own style when
> coping with anxiety or a potential
> threat? Are you more inclined to
> avoid and try to forget it or pay
> close attention and learn what
> you can about it?

buying an article of clothing. How many options do you want to consider before deciding? The stakes may be higher when the uncertainty is distressing. In considering a medical procedure like surgery, some people want to know all the details ahead of time, perhaps even watching a video demonstration, whereas others don't want to know: "Just put me out and do it."[2]

Predicting the Future

One basis for anticipating the future is what you yourself have experienced in the past. Hope based on experience is a fundamental part of learning. The Russian physiologist Ivan Pavlov won a Nobel prize in 1904 for demonstrating classical conditioning in an experiment with dogs: If he consistently rang a bell right before feeding them, the dogs would soon begin to salivate when just hearing the dinner bell. If you have had household pets, you have probably experienced their excited behavior in anticipation of food, a homecoming, or going outside. Based on experience, we develop expectations about how particular people are going to behave, and we come to anticipate, even rely on, their consistency. When someone has been dependably kind to you, it is natural to hope, even take for granted, that they will continue to do so. You have tamed each other. A rebuke from such a person can come as a shock and be especially painful. We have a responsibility to be gentle with those whom we have tamed.[3]

Apart from your personal experience, there are mathematical probabilities based on data. Given all the available evidence, what is the likelihood of various possible outcomes? Probabilities are one way to judge how *realistic* hope is. Sometimes the odds are straightforward. On a single coin toss, the chances of its coming up heads would be 50 percent. Getting 10 heads in a row is possible but highly unlikely; in fact it's less than one chance in a thousand. Now suppose you have just tossed a coin in the air nine times, and all nine times it came up heads. Assuming that it's an unbiased coin, what are the chances that the next time it will be tails? The answer of course is still 50 percent. You might expect that now tails is long overdue after nine heads, but in fact the chance remains 50/50. The prior tosses have no effect at all on the outcome of the 10th toss. It is still a random event. The classic gambler's fallacy is believing that a chance event will be more (or less) likely to occur based on the outcome of previous chance events.

Guessing what *people* are going to do is a lot more complex, although our behavior is actually more predictable than we might wish to believe.[4] In contrast to coin tosses, a tried-and-true psychological principle is that past behavior predicts future behavior. At least in a similar situation, people are likely (though not certain) to behave as they have before. If you serve on a jury, you may be called upon to decide beyond a reasonable doubt, based on the evidence, whether someone committed a crime of which they are accused, and prior offenses might be considered if the judge allows it. Parole boards try to anticipate how dangerous to society an offender might be if released. Yet it is very difficult to foretell future dangerousness, even though such predictions are often used to influence vital decisions in criminal justice systems, including in capital punishment cases.[5] In a 2017 position statement on assessing the risk for violence, the American Psychiatric Association acknowledged that "While psychiatrists can often identify circumstances associated with an increased likelihood of violent behavior, they cannot predict dangerousness with definitive accuracy."

One problem is that when trying to predict relatively infrequent events, most of the time you probably will be wrong. Even if as many as one-third of prior offenders will commit a new crime, a prediction of recidivism will be wrong two times out of three. Another obstacle is that definitions of dangerousness can be vague.[6] Predicting the recurrence of a specific offense such as drunk driving can be somewhat more accurate when using objective risk factors instead of personal judgment.[7] There is a long history of studies showing that actuarial prediction from objective data is more accurate than human expert judgment.[8] Even when an artificial intelligence system "looks over the shoulder" of clinicians to determine how they make judgments, the machine will then be more accurate in predicting future cases than is the clinician from whom it learned.[9] How can this be? The machine applies the abstracted decision rules with complete consistency, uninfluenced by subjective factors, sympathy, or what it had for breakfast. Apart from accuracy, judgments about dangerousness are also ethically complex, balancing individual human considerations against social safety.[10] How serious was the offense? What *is* an acceptable level of risk?

Under conditions of uncertainty we tend to form impressions about what is likely to happen and then make decisions based on those guesses.[11] Human judgment in such matters is notoriously flawed by cognitive biases.[12] For example, first impressions and decision making can be influenced by automatic mental processes that operate below consciousness. One obvious example (though less apparent to us when we're in the midst of forming impressions) is that we tend to be biased toward people who are tall and attractive. In a majority of U.S. presidential elections, the taller candidate has won. Malcolm Gladwell dubbed this the "Warren Harding error," after the tall, good-looking candidate who in 1920 was elected to the height of power in the United States.[13] Harding looked downright presidential but proved to be one of the most incompetent occupants of the White House. This is one example of the *halo effect,* a well-demonstrated bias in our perception and judgment. Having some positive or negative information about someone tends to generalize to their unknown characteristics.[14] We may overlook or not even see negative aspects of someone we like or love, and the opposite is also true: We discount positive attributes of people whom we dislike. First impressions can also be biased by recent experience. Estimates of divorce rates are affected by how easily examples come to your mind, and recent mood influences the favorability of judgments.[15] People's predictions about the weather differ depending on whether they're in a bright or gloomy mood.

Indeed, hope itself biases our judgment,[16] and so does fear.[17] Our optimism about whether something will occur is influenced by many factors. We constantly pay attention to any new information about the probability of happenings, even in ordinary conversations. Suppose you ask a friend to do something, perhaps to help you move to a new abode. You will watch and listen carefully to how the person responds to your request, to the spoken words as well as to facial expression, gestures, and tone of voice. Why? Because they contain information about how likely you are to get the help.

How might each of the following responses to a request influence your hopefulness? Can you feel your hope rising or falling with each of them?

I'd like to help you.

I might be able to help you.

I'm willing to help you.

I wish I could help you.

You probably are going to need help.

I hope that I can help you.

I remember you've helped me before.

I will help you.

I promise I'll help.

Such statements offer clues about how hopeful you should be that the person is going to help.[18] They also open the way for some negotiation toward an agreement. When you feel hopeful or would like to, you are weighing how real your expectation is, how likely it is to come true. Your guesses fluctuate as you receive new information like the statements above. The prospects you perceive will land somewhere between zero and certainty on a mental scale something like this:

Impossible	Unlikely	Possible	Probable	Sure Thing

Hope and Prognosis

In health care, hope is called *prognosis*—expectations about the future based on what is known about the condition. Diagnoses themselves may impact hope. It can be comforting to have a name for what you're suffering, giving you a sense that at least someone understands what it is, as if knowing the name of a demon can help to exorcise it. At the same time, a diagnostic label may convey a sense of doom, depending on what we know and believe about the condition. For many years people avoided even saying the word *cancer*, and still it can evoke fear. Contrary to public impressions of continual decline, most people diagnosed with alcohol/drug addiction or schizophrenia improve significantly over time,[19] and hope itself can contribute to their recovery.[20] Early in its history, the COVID-19 pandemic prompted worldwide fear and dramatic changes in behavior. As vaccines and effective treatments became available, fear diminished and so did the use of protective measures.

With long-term conditions where recurrences are normal, how does a setback affect hope? Again it has to do with expectations. With a chronic illness like asthma, hypertension, or depression, symptom recurrences are normal. It is not expected that a patient will *never* again have an asthmatic episode, high blood pressure, or depressed mood. In my own field of addiction treatment a recurrence of symptoms is also quite common, but ironically it is often interpreted as a failure ("relapse") that can undermine hope.[21] Thinking in such black-and-white terms is misleading. In a study with over 8,000 people who had been treated for alcohol use disorders, we first counted those who had completely abstained from alcohol for 12 months or more.[22] By that standard, the average success rate of treatment was 24 percent, but what about all the rest who on a statistical survival curve would be classified as relapsed? For the remaining three-fourths of people their drinking had decreased by 87 percent during the year after treatment and their alcohol-related troubles by 60 percent. For any chronic illness like diabetes, that result would be considered a remarkable success: 24 percent complete remission, and for the rest an 87 percent reduction in the primary symptom. No one even computes "success rates" when treating diabetes or heart disease. A good outcome of treatment over time is to have fewer and less severe symptoms that are separated by gradually longer periods of remission.

I devoted much of my career to developing and evaluating treatments for common recurring psychological conditions, such as depression, anxiety, and addictions. When people seek treatment of such illnesses for themselves or a loved one, they often have little idea where to begin. Searching for help on the web (or, once upon a time, in the phone book) can yield a bewildering array of options. My own recommendation has been to seek treatments that are most strongly supported by scientific evidence, though this is itself a complex question.[23] Most people thus tend to rely on their care providers to keep up with the scientific literature.

Nevertheless, our desires influence the evidence we attend to and believe. The ever-present cognitive confirmation bias is that it's more comfortable to hear information confirming what we already believe and to discount inconvenient truths. I was lectured this week by a cigarette smoker with impassioned convictions about which kind of sea salt is healthiest and the importance of using sugar rather than artificial sweeteners. We readily forgive our own inconsistencies. At conference refreshment tables I pick up a diet soda and a chocolate chip cookie with some vague assurance that they cancel each other out.

False Hope

What is false about hope?[24] From the rational perspective of probability it does make sense to talk about *false* hope. There are many situations in which, based on the current evidence, there's very little reason for confidence, and hope can be said to be unrealistic from a statistical vantage point. Hucksters offer enticing false images of hope to promote products, services, or speculative investments in the absence of legitimate evidence.[25] Bernie Madoff made off with investors' billions in the largest Ponzi scheme on record, and

Elizabeth Holmes built her $9 billion Theranos corporation on the fraudulent but enticing promise of being able to perform comprehensive serum assays from a single drop of blood.

The concept of being "in denial" suggests holding on to unrealistic hope. Refusing to accept a shocking reality is a common, even normal, reaction to new information such as the diagnosis of a terminal illness.[26] It can take a while to get used to a new reality. Hearing about alternative treatments can bolster hope for those with life-threatening conditions.[27] A desperate desire for hope can render suffering people vulnerable to charlatans who market pathways to hope without sound scientific evidence.

In another sense, however, there is no such thing as false hope. Predictive rationality based on evidence is but one facet of the rich human experience of hope that can also be a feeling, an intuition, a longing, a conviction, or a matter of trust and faith. Who then is to say that someone's hope is wrong or misguided? Things seem impossible until they're not: the right of women to vote, peace in Northern Ireland, and same-sex marriage. We never know for sure which hopes are false, including our own.[28] The 148th Kentucky Derby was run at Churchill Downs in May of 2022. The lead horse changed several times during a fast-paced race, and those who had put their money down on Rich Strike to win were betting against 80-to-1 odds with little rational reason for hope. Yet this last-minute long-shot entry in the 20-horse field came from far behind and ran on the rail to one of the biggest upsets in derby history. Sometimes the seemingly impossible does happen.

The truth that hope can endure and sustain us for better or worse against all odds is found at the heart of countless stories, both fictional and actual.[29] In Melville's *Moby Dick*, Captain Ahab persists in hopeful pursuit of a white whale to the doom of himself and all but one of his crew. Heroic ocean survival is the subject of Hemingway's story *The Old Man and the Sea*, and it also happens in real life. Attempting a 4,000-mile sail from Tahiti to San Diego, Tami Oldham Ashcraft awoke at sea after being knocked unconscious from a head injury during a hurricane, her fiancé missing and apparently drowned. With masts broken and sails destroyed, she drifted alone for 41 days before being spotted and rescued off Hawaii.[30] The Mexican fisherman José Salvador Alvarenga survived for an incredible 438 days drifting for 6,000 miles in the Pacific Ocean after his small craft's motor was destroyed in a storm.[31]

> Would you bet on an expensive treatment with a 5 percent cure rate and life-threatening risks of its own when faced with an illness that was almost sure to end your life? What would be the "rational" choice? It's the stuff of medical TV shows and also of real-life hospitals.

False Hopelessness

Just as hope can be unfounded from a rational perspective, so can hopelessness. A long-studied personality predisposition called *locus of control* is whether you tend to believe that what happens to you is generally determined by your own actions (internal locus) or by factors beyond your control, such as fate or luck (external locus).[32] People with an external locus of control are less likely to engage in protective measures, such as buying disaster insurance,[33] accepting vaccinations,[34] or even taking shelter during a tornado warning.[35] Those with an external locus are also less likely to adopt long-term environmental protection practices, such as recycling,[36] soil conservation,[37] or efforts to reduce global warming.[38] Low-hope people are more likely to take risks with financial decisions,[39] substance use,[40] and sexual behavior.[41] In essence, the underlying belief is that "There's nothing I can do," "What I do won't make any difference," or "Whatever will be will be."

There is a self-defeating aspect of such fatalistic beliefs. Failing to take protective action invites the natural consequences, thus confirming powerlessness as a self-fulfilling prophecy.[42] The opposite risk is persisting too long in efforts to change what is genuinely immutable. In his famous "serenity prayer" from the early 1930s Reinhold Niebuhr wrote: "Give us courage to change what must be changed, serenity to accept what cannot be helped, and the insight to know the one from the other." The prayer was subsequently reworded by putting "serenity" first, and it continues to be widely used in 12-step groups, such as Alcoholics Anonymous, in this more familiar form:

> God, grant me the serenity to accept the things I cannot
>   change,
> courage to change the things I can,
> and wisdom to know the difference.

The prayer seeks to steer a healthy course between false hope and false hopelessness.

A theme that runs through this book is that hope not only anticipates but also shapes the future. People with higher hope are more likely to have subsequent accomplishments as concrete as athletic achievement and a higher college grade-point average. A person's level of hope predicts their actual performance above and beyond their natural ability as rated by teachers.[43] Estimating likelihood is only one facet of hope. It is natural to consider the odds, but human hope has more dimensions in spite of the odds.

What Hope Is Not

Finally, let's consider some things that hope is not, at least not necessarily. First, hope is not denial, refusing to recognize reality. Often hope persists despite the odds, in witness against how things are. To forgive does not require you to forget what happened or to say that it was all right. If you did forget or really thought that what the person did was OK, there would be no need to forgive. Forgiveness is chosen with full awareness, often with hope for a better future.[44] Late in the Vietnam War a few celebrations were organized to mark the end of the war even though the end seemed to be nowhere in sight. They were not held because the participants falsely believed the war to be ended. They were living as if it was over, as a testament of hope that it would be. Hope is not denial of current reality.

Second, hope is not the same as acceptance, acquiescence, or inaction. Saying "I just hope that . . ." may connote passivity, but not necessarily so.[45] To the contrary, hope can undergird persistent efforts toward change, and such action is itself a form of hoping (Chapter 8). The promise of hope is not in the presence of one particular form but in the varieties that are available to the human spirit.

Finally, hope is not necessarily evidence based. Although statistical evidence can be grounds for encouragement, it is only one factor that comes into play when we face uncertainty. For some people and in some situations, probability may be the primary consideration: What are my chances? Yet for others, even the slightest glimmer of possibility is sufficient. "If there is *any* chance, I'll go for it." People buy lottery tickets, where the likelihood of winning a jackpot is one in hundreds of millions. We also vary in our tolerance for risk taking. Some people are averse to even infinitesimal dangers, such as being attacked by a shark while wading or swimming along an ocean shoreline. Others play chicken with life-threatening games or habits. Probability is but one consideration, one facet of the fascinating diamond of hope. I have sometimes lamented a child's life choices, and I know well the principle that past behavior is the best predictor of future behavior. Yet my paternal hope is not grounded in a *belief* or even a *prediction* that the future will be different. Even when all current indications are to the contrary, my hope envisions the possibility of a different future. It is to this third source of hope that we turn next.

TAKING IT PERSONALLY: PROBABILITY

- What sources of information do you usually rely on to know what is happening around you in your community, country, or world? Of all the possible ways now available to get such information, why do you happen to trust those particular sources?

- How do you decide when something might be unrealistic or a false hope? When in your own life has someone told you that a hope of yours was unrealistic? How did that affect you at the time?

- Which mistake are you more likely to make: (1) to give up on something that you actually could change or (2) to keep on trying to change something that you actually cannot change?

CHAPTER 4

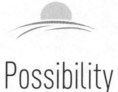

Possibility

What after all has maintained the human race on
this old globe despite all the calamities of nature
and all the tragic failings of mankind, if not faith
in new possibilities, and courage to advocate them?
—JANE ADDAMS

Once you choose hope, anything's possible.
—CHRISTOPHER REEVE

She seemed to be a hopeless case. As a young child, Annie was left nearly blind from a bacterial eye disease. Her mother died of tuberculosis when she was only 8 years old, after which her father, unable to cope, abandoned the family. She and her younger brother, Jimmy, were consigned to a notorious poorhouse for the sick and insane, where Jimmy died 4 months later. Annie endured four painful and unsuccessful eye surgeries and finally at age 14 was sent off to a school for the blind, where several more operations partially restored her vision. She graduated first in her class, became a teacher, and her very first student was a 7-year-old blind and deaf girl named Helen Keller. Annie Sullivan believed that it would be possible for Helen to learn and communicate, and she undertook the demanding work required to make it happen. With

time, Helen not only learned how to communicate but
became a famous writer, lecturer, and advocate for disability rights. At age 35, Annie suffered a stroke and was
herself left completely blind. She would later be called
"the miracle worker" in a play of that name produced for
television, Broadway, and film. She died at age 70 with
Helen Keller holding her hand, and Annie's ashes are
interred at the National Cathedral in Washington.[1]

To base your hope on probability and history is to see life only as
it has been. Hope sees the prospect of what could be and is not yet.
Faithful fans of a struggling sports team base their enthusiasm not
on statistics but rather on envisioned possibility. They can imagine the nascent or fumbling team they love eventually winning the
World Cup in soccer or the immodestly named World Series in
U.S. baseball, and sometimes it does happen. Love sees what is as
yet unrealized potential.[2] Anne Sullivan realized what her young
student Helen *could* be. It is the same transforming vision of Don
Quixote, who perceived a peasant girl Aldonza to be the noble Lady
Dulcinea. Is it really madness? "Maddest of all," Quixote says, is "to
see life as it is and not as it should be."[3]

Seeing Possibility

Broadly speaking, there are two important elements that influence
a person's motivation to act: why and how. The *why* component is
that there is good enough reason for action and change; it is a sufficiently *important* matter. It might be a hope for positive gain and
improvement or a fear of loss and negative outcome to be avoided.
Yet the need for change can be clear, even urgent, but no action is

taken unless there's also a belief that it's possible, that there is a *how*. Hope requires both desire and possibility.

On November 20, 1983, the ABC television network aired a new film, *The Day After*, that dramatized the aftermath of a nuclear war. It was a national event; more than 100 million people tuned in during the initial broadcast, making it one of the most-watched events ever. Immediately after the alarming movie, ABC aired a distinguished panel discussion hosted by Ted Koppel, who repeatedly asked the panelists, "Is there anything Americans can do to prevent this? What can an individual do?"

All the panelists agreed that nuclear war would be a catastrophe, and astrophysicist Carl Sagan said that the reality of it would actually be far worse than had been portrayed in the film. Defense Secretary Robert McNamara recommended supporting his administration's current nuclear policy, and General Brent Scowcroft warned that the current nuclear deterrent was insufficient. Secretary of State George Shultz argued that the government should reduce the number of nuclear weapons, while national security advisor Henry Kissinger countered that more weapons keep us safer. Author William F. Buckley Jr. accused the filmmaker of trying to undermine America's defenses. Holocaust survivor Elie Wiesel said he felt scared and helpless and agreed with Buckley that pacifism is dangerous. Nobody offered a single hopeful suggestion for individual action. In other words, the film spoke loudly to the *importance* of the issue but was immediately followed by a message that there was nothing individuals could do about it. I suspect that had the film been followed by a practical suggestion or two for what ordinary people could do to have an impact, it might have triggered a movement.

Scare tactics suffer a similar fate in health care, whether it's a lecture on the dangers of drug use or a stern medical caution about weight gain and heart disease. The importance of action must be paired with at least the perception that change is possible. It does no good to convince someone that a situation is dire without the possibility of making a difference. Many people see global warming as an imminent threat but seem to believe there is nothing they can really do about it. Scare tactics are less likely to inspire behavior change than to prompt defensiveness that in conversations can appear as arguing, challenging, discounting, interrupting, or simply ignoring. Remember that fear is an opposite of hope. Confronted by threat without hope, people tend to shut down and stop listening.

What is often missed is the cumulative effect of small changes. It's the mistake of doing nothing because it's only possible for you to do a little. Even during the COVID-19 pandemic in 2021 in the United States alone, 60 million adults gave over 4 billion hours of volunteer time with various organizations, resulting in huge economic and social benefits.[4] Beyond the collective impact of individual efforts, *doing* something positive to address adversity also benefits the doer's health and well-being. A clear example is volunteering time with service organizations. People who volunteer significant time experience better mood, optimism, hope, and purpose in life, less depression and loneliness, and decreased risk of mortality.[5]

> Where do you (or could you) make small contributions toward larger changes that matter to you?

Seeing possibility raises your vision beyond the present reality. Hope may be dismissed as unrealistic, but Richard Rohr suggests another way of seeing: "We can call hope true realism, because hope takes seriously all the many possibilities that fill the moment. Hope sees all the alternatives."[6]

Seeing Possibility in Others

If love is blind, then how does it happen that falling in love can turn into the long-term satisfying relationship for which the partners hope? Lovers do tend to idealize each other. When infatuated, we focus on, exaggerate, and fantasize about each other's good qualities and are inclined to overlook faults, at least for the time being. As invariably imperfect people, wouldn't that just be a setup for inevitable disappointment and unhappiness?

As it turns out, our positive perceptions of and hopes for those we love can be amazingly resilient over time. Seeing an imperfect partner in idealized ways can create stable relationships. Happier and more enduring relationships are those in which people think more highly of their partners than the partners think of themselves. Furthermore, thinking highly of your spouse can actually improve your partner's own self-esteem.[7] Hope might also improve reality as time passes; people may try to live up to admiring perceptions and thereby confirm them (see Chapter 2). It is essentially projecting your hope onto someone and giving them the benefit of the doubt. When in doubt, hope! Sometimes we can see things into being.

I don't know who decided long ago that a working-class boy in a small Pennsylvania coal-mining town should be placed in the college-preparatory track; apparently they saw possibility in me. I *do* know and remember the names of teachers who took it from there during secondary school and college. There was Mary Duncan, who schooled us in Latin and made it fun. We sang a Latin translation of "Jingle Bells,"[8] then later in her German class our final exam was listening to and translating a popular song.[9] In freshman English it was Gertrude Madden, who took the time needed to mark up our essays in detail, helping countless college students learn how to write more effectively—something that I would later try to do for my own students. Our formidable choirmaster Walter McIver listened to my quavering voice, told me that he liked what he heard, and through spirited coaching gave me a gift that would last a lifetime. When I went in to confess my emerging agnosticism, the college chaplain, Paul Neufer, told me, "That's a good place to grow from!" and so it was. In many individual conversations the psychology department chair, George Shortess, listened respectfully to my young ideas and gently encouraged me toward my eventual profession. The Irish poet James J. McAuley heard a meter hidden within my poor approximations to poetry and taught me to prize spare writing and speech. I am so grateful to these mentors who saw possibilities in me of which I had been unaware. They perceived what I could be and were patient in calling it forth, not in a hurry for me to change and grow, but happy for me to do so in my own time and way.

Hidden possibility also runs through a well-known biblical story of a woman captured in the very act of adultery, which at the time was punishable by immediate death from stoning. Howard Thurman described her being taken to Rabbi Jesus for judgment.

> He met the woman where she was, and he treated her as if she were already where she now willed to be. In dealing with her he "believed" her into the fulfillment of her possibilities. He stirred her confidence into activity. He placed a crown over her head which for the rest of her life she would keep trying to grow tall enough to wear.[10]

The rabbi's approach was transformation rather than retribution. He also saw a possibility in the bystanders who were already eagerly picking up rocks. "Let the one among you who has never sinned throw the first stone at her." Then he sat down and waited patiently as they all walked away one by one, *beginning with the oldest*.[11] Hope as perceived possibility can literally bring out the best in others.

Believing in Possibility: The Placebo Effect

He came to the clinic complaining of an odd obsession, and perhaps because of my interest in addictions he was referred to me. Raul was a professional artist who used a form of meditation to quiet his mind and tap into the deep creative river within him. For several months, however, whenever he had entered this meditative state he encountered an intrusive image: the face of a man who was a stranger to him. The face was always the same, not particularly threatening, but just there "in the upper-left-hand corner" of the blank canvas behind his eyelids. He found it terribly distressing and distracting, and it was seriously interfering with his creative productivity. "I think it might help if you hypnotized me," he said. I had been trained in clinical hypnosis but also knew the research literature at the time on treating obsessions, so I explained my understanding that there was no good scientific evidence that hypnosis would help him. For 2 months or so I tried a variety of evidence-based treatment strategies, all to no avail. Finally, in desperation, I hypnotized him with a classic trance induction and a posthypnotic suggestion that the obsession would be gone. He called me 4 days later. "Doc! It's amazing! He's completely gone! Thanks—I don't need to come in anymore." And I never saw him again.[12] *Raul reminded me to listen to what people believe will help them.*

Clear evidence of the power of hope as possibility is found within the placebo effect in healing. When given a treatment that they are told will help them, people often get better. Particularly in pain relief, placebos are substantially more effective than no treatment at all. The effect is more than just natural healing with the passage of time. An inert placebo is often more effective than no pill even when patients know that what they are taking might be a placebo.[13] So significant is this effect that new medications are required to be tested against a placebo control in which neither the doctor nor the patient knows which is which. What's going on here?

Placebo relief of pain is real; people receiving placebo medication (containing no active ingredients) report reduced pain and show corresponding reductions of brain activation in areas related to pain and anxiety. A medication (naloxone) that blocks the pain-relieving effects of opiate drugs like morphine also reduces the effectiveness of placebos, suggesting that they work in part through the body's natural endorphins that also use the opiate receptors. Pain-alleviating drugs are twice as effective when patients know they are receiving them, as compared with the same doses administered without the person's knowledge. Patients who are warned about possible side effects of a placebo are more likely to experience them.[14] Furthermore, people who are told that they will receive a powerful pain-relieving medication show much greater pain relief with a placebo than do those who are told that they might be receiving a placebo.[15]

Expectation effects are not limited to medications. Other placebo research has studied what happens when people are given beverages that they are told do or don't contain alcohol. In a clever four-group "balanced-placebo" study design,[16] people are given beverages with or without alcohol and are told that it does or does not contain alcohol. When believing (incorrectly) that they are drinking alcohol (in comparison to anticipating no alcohol content), people drink more, become more sociable, less anxious, more sexually aroused, and more aggressive. Their expectations about alcohol's effects come true without the alcohol. In contrast, the impairing effects of alcohol on memory, mental functioning, and ability to perform physical tasks happen whether or not people know that there is alcohol in the beverage they are drinking.[17]

Now here's another puzzle. Recent research has questioned whether it's really mental expectations that are at work in the potent effect of placebos. Open-label studies give placebos to patients who *know* that they are taking placebos. It even says "placebo" right on the bottle of pills. Wouldn't this undo the effect?; or said another way, does the placebo effect depend on deception? Professor Ted Kaptchuk at Harvard Medical School has been using open-label placebos to treat patients with chronic conditions that defy medical alleviation: migraine headaches, depression, allergies, fatigue, lower back pain, and irritable bowel syndrome.[18] These are patients who are unimpressed by white coats and medical degrees. They expressly do *not* anticipate being helped; their long, disappointing experience with doctors and treatments has led them to expect failure. People in these studies are told truthfully that well-controlled studies have shown the powerful effects of placebos on their condition and that it happens automatically. They don't have to believe that the treatment will work, but it is critical that they take the pills twice a day. Those given open-label placebos show a reduction of symptoms and suffering. Reviewing subsequent interviews with patients, Kaptchuk concluded that "patients did not endorse positive expectations, but rather spoke of something they called *hope*," which he called "a lifejacket against despair, a disposition that allows patients to face illness and maintain a semblance of a life."[19] Expectation, he said, relies on *past* experience, whereas hope is open to *new* experience.

Neither are placebo effects limited to drugs. A German physician, Franz Anton Mesmer, claimed to be able to cure a broad array of maladies by manipulating patients' "animal magnetism" through various rituals. His cures were so widespread, and he grew so popular and successful in Paris that the king of France appointed two commissions to examine Mesmer's claims, one of the first-recorded investigations of scientific fraud. The Faculty of Medicine commission was chaired by a visiting American scientist named Benjamin Franklin, who devised some clever experiments. Mesmer and his disciples claimed to be able to magnetize patients or objects without touching them, and Franklin's commission anticipated by 2 centuries the balanced placebo design mentioned earlier. Using blindfolds and curtains, Mesmer's staff would "magnetize" patients with or without their awareness, and patients would also be told they were being magnetized whether or not a mesmerist was present. They further had mesmerists magnetize certain trees within a walled garden and then released patients into the garden to choose a tree to hug. In his thorough report,[20] Franklin demonstrated that there was no relationship between whether patients had been "magnetized" and their symptomatic improvement. Mesmer was disgraced and driven from Paris. Franklin noted that dramatic healings *did* happen, but not because of magnetism. In his 1785 report he mused that:

> This new agent might be no other than the imagination itself, whose power is as extensive as it is little known. . . . The imagination of sick persons has unquestionably a very frequent and considerable share in the cure of their diseases. . . . In [the

physical world] as well as religion, [we] are saved by faith . . . under the genial influence of hope. Hope is an essential constituent of human life.[21]

In counseling and psychotherapy research there is no direct parallel to a double-blind placebo, precisely because the therapist always *knows* what treatment is being provided. In medication trials the drug can be administered in a way that neither patient nor provider knows what is in the capsule, but this is not possible in psychotherapy. If therapists believe the treatment to be ineffective, their expectations influence client outcomes.[22] It matters that providers believe in the treatment they are delivering.[23] Of course, it's possible to evaluate a treatment that the therapist believes in but is arbitrarily regarded by the researcher to be inert, in which case investigator bias is a concern. In the mesmerism study the efficacy of the method was in doubt, though apparently not to the patients. As Franklin himself observed, "His cures were numerous and of the most astonishing nature."[24] In the treed garden patients did find relief from their suffering, just not for the reason that Mesmer proposed. The hope of both patients and their providers was sufficient to yield beneficial results.

Possible Futures

A fundamental aspect of hope is an openness to possible futures. Howard Thurman observed that "in the absence of all hope ambition dies, and the very self is weakened, corroded."[25] An absence of hope forecloses on the future.

Certain life events may change your vision of possible futures. Prolonged stress or a diagnosis of advanced cancer can shatter the taken-for-granted quality of life and narrow the horizon of alterna-tives.[26] People may mourn the loss of future options and treasure what was once assumed. On the other hand, receiving treatment can foster hope for better life, and having a teacher who believes in you can open up possible futures.

Personality also matters. One individual difference with implications for possibilities is a dimension from Jungian psychol-ogy known as *sensing-intuiting*.[27] Sens-ing people are realists. They prefer to rely on, attend to, and enjoy the wit-ness of their senses—seeing, hearing, touching, smelling, and tasting. They trust the here-and-now and notice what is right there in front of them. Those at the other end of the spectrum prefer to experience the world through intuition and insight and may have a hard time explaining how they know things. They prefer more to dream and imagine, to see possibilities, and they may live more in the future than in the present. If they are living together in a house while it is being built, the sensing person will notice all the details of what still needs to be done, whereas the intuiting person happily perceives the house as it will be in the future. Those at opposite ends of this personality dimension may have a hard time understanding each other because they literally experience different realities.[28] They need and balance each other's perspective.

> What are one or two possible futures that you once considered for yourself but wound up following a different path?

Complementary differences in emphasis on past and present reality versus hope for a better future are also found in justice sys-tems. Retributive justice focuses on punishment and revenge for past offenses. A restorative approach emphasizes future possibilities for transformation and relationship in corrections, education, and responding to social injustice.[29]

Perceived Influence

One component of hope as possibility has to do with your perceived ability to influence what will happen in the future. Do you think that this situation, problem, or person is malleable in general or even by you personally?[30] Hope is important, for example, in conflict resolution. Willingness to compromise and work for peace is affected by whether people regard a conflict to be resolvable or intractable.[31] Believing that there is something you can do to influence the future matters.

Here's a simple example from research on stressful situations. Volunteers in a series of experiments were exposed to painfully loud noise or electric shocks. Some of the volunteers were given a button that they could press to turn off the noise or shock in the event that it became intolerable, whereas others were offered no such button.[32] It actually didn't matter whether the button worked because no one ever pressed it—they had been encouraged not to unless absolutely necessary. People who had an escape button—something they could do—were more tolerant, less physically distressed, and more able to concentrate on the tasks they were asked to perform.[33] Believing there is something you can do to control or at least influence a stressful situation makes a significant difference. In a study of brief psychotherapy, two-thirds of client satisfaction was related to a single questionnaire item: "The counselor encouraged me to believe that I could improve my situation."[34]

Often in my own research it was the unexpected findings that were most important. In seeking better ways to help problem drinkers we sometimes compared reductions in drinking for people who were given immediate treatment versus those placed on a waiting list to receive the same treatment later. Those put on a waiting list showed no apparent change until we had treated them.[35] This outcome seemed somewhat odd because just to get into the study they had expressed concern about their alcohol use, undergone a thorough evaluation, reported distressing levels of drinking, and requested help, all of which might be expected in themselves to raise their awareness and encourage trying out some efforts for change. Yet there was no change at all. In another study[36] we added a comparison group who received just one session in which we sent them home with a self-help book,[37] encouraging them to follow the instructions. Other participants in the same study were given immediate counseling using the same methods described in the self-help book, and still another group of problem drinkers were told they were on a 10-week waiting list for treatment. Once again, those on the waiting list showed no change at all in their drinking, while those given immediate treatment cut their alcohol use in half. The less expected finding was that people randomly assigned to work on their own using the self-help book reduced their drinking by two-thirds. What was the difference? Those on the waiting list were given the implicit message that there was nothing they could do until we would treat them. They actually did what we told them to do: they waited. In contrast, those in the self-help condition were asked to proceed on their own following the guidelines we provided; they were told there was something they could do, and they did it. I now believe that waiting lists can be harmful by suggesting helplessness.[38] Better, when possible, to give people something effective to do rather than waiting.

Seeing a possible pathway forward is both a source and a product of hope.[39] More hopeful people persist in finding ways to reach their goals, even and especially when a planned path is obstructed. They view setbacks as challenges rather than failures, giving themselves positive messages like "I'll find a way to get this done!"[40] Hope encourages them to channel their concerns into individual or collective action rather than resorting to denial, distraction, or other ways to reduce emotional distress.[41]

So beyond making judgments about how likely something is to happen (Chapter 3), hope also extends to seeing possibilities in the future, in yourself and in others. In perceiving and pursuing possibilities, the seemingly improbable can happen because, at least in part, what you see is what you get. You don't just see things as they are. You also see things as *you* are, influenced by your history, personality, mood, and expectations.[42] Perceiving possibility prompts trying, and these attempts in turn can change things and change you as well. Not every wish comes true, but seeing possibility can make it more likely to happen.

Desire, probability, and possibility are all potent varieties of hope that can differ in strength over time. When reflecting on a particular hoped-for goal, your mind may flit from one of these facets to another. What is the evidence so far? What might be possible? What do you really want? Another facet of hope is optimism, which is a more stable attribute of personality or character and is the subject of the next chapter.

TAKING IT PERSONALLY: POSSIBILITY

- How does feeling hopeful and seeing possibilities affect you?

- Who in your life saw possibilities in you that you didn't know you had and helped to bring them out in you?

- What life experiences have opened up or closed down your perceived possible futures?

CHAPTER 5

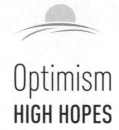

Optimism
HIGH HOPES

All shall be well, and all shall be well, and all manner
of things shall be exceeding well.
—Julian of Norwich[1]

A pessimist sees the difficulty in every opportunity;
an optimist sees the opportunity in every difficulty.
—Sir Winston Churchill

We had never met these strangers who would be our children. We had seen them only briefly on the evening news during a weekly feature called "Wednesday's Child," named from a line in a 19th-century nursery rhyme that "Wednesday's child is full of woe." The TV reporter had taken Lillian and Richard to a pet store, where they longingly cuddled puppies who were also in need of a good home. At ages 9 and 8 they had already suffered more than a lifetime's share of woe. Now, after a year of screening and qualifying to be adoptive parents, we waited in the social worker's outer office, unsure what to expect or say on this first face-to-face encounter. We needn't have worried about how to greet them. The inner door opened, and Lillian came bounding toward us exclaiming, "Hi, Mom! Hi, Dad!"

Every kind of hope is an experience of expectation, even when based on statistical prediction. Thus far we have considered three facets of hope: desire, probability, and possibility. Sometimes hope is specific and situational: You hope that something in particular will happen. In contrast, the kind of hope discussed in this chapter is more like a personality characteristic or character trait—an enduring disposition to look on the bright side, expect the good, and give the benefit of the doubt. People who typically show such high hopefulness across time and situations are called *optimistic*.

Optimism is different from having particular hopes. Optimists tend to expect that in life things will usually turn out for the best, at least in the long run.[2] They have positive thoughts and feelings about the future in general without necessarily seeing a way for it to happen.[3] Questionnaires designed to measure optimism include items like "When the future is in doubt, I usually expect the best," and "I generally anticipate more good than bad things to happen."[4] The popular 1988 song by Bobby McFerrin, "Don't Worry, Be Happy" expresses this view. So does the often-quoted perspective at the head of this chapter from the 14th-century mystic Julian or Juliana of Norwich, author of the first book known to have been written in English by a woman.

Like hope more generally, optimism can be passive, active, or both. A wishful or *passive optimism* sees hope in the efforts of others and in forces beyond oneself, as with optimism about the weather or hopefulness on the day of an election. In contrast, *active optimism* recognizes a personal role that you can play in bringing about a desired outcome or preventing unwanted events, such as in hoping to earn a good grade in a course or to avoid having a heart attack.[5] Health promotion efforts encourage active optimism, managing your own behavior to prevent illness and improve your long-term well-being. An optimistic perspective can embrace both active and passive elements—some that are within your control and others that are not.

Optimism is one of a cluster of four interrelated personal traits that together have been called *positivity* or *psychological capital*. The other three characteristics of positivity are hope more generally, resilience, and agency or efficacy.[6] *Resilience* is the ability to rebound from, adapt to, and persist despite adversity.[7] You are unlikely to succeed without trying, and making attempts is a product of your belief in the possibility of success. *Agency* is the belief "that good events can be made more likely and bad events less [likely] by appropriate actions on the part of the individual"—in other words, that you can produce desired results by what you do.[8] The belief that one's own efforts can be fruitful is strong motivation to take action. In the children's story *The Little Engine That Could*, the title character's persistent effort is maintained by the chant "I think I can, I think I can." Dolores Huerta's simple phrase "Si, se puede" (Yes, it's possible, or Yes, we can) became the empowering motto of the United Farm Workers in 1972.[9] These characteristics of positivity can be developed in both individuals and organizations.[10]

Benefits of Optimism

Optimism is easily belittled as unrealistic or naïve. The term *narapoia* was coined as an opposite delusion from paranoia—an irrational belief that people are actually plotting to do you good.[11]

Although optimism might be regarded as detrimental, there is a good deal of evidence to the contrary.

In psychological research, optimism is one of the personality characteristics most consistently associated with a variety of happy outcomes. A summary of this large body of research concluded that "hope and optimism (or at least the absence of their opposites) are associated with all manner of desirable outcomes: positive mood and good morale; perseverance and effective problem solving; academic, athletic, military, occupational, and political success; popularity; good health; and even long life and freedom from trauma."[12] Among the documented correlates of optimism are:

- A greater subjective sense of well-being[13]
- Better social adjustment to stressful events and life transitions[14]
- Fewer immature defense mechanisms such as denial, projection, and magical thinking[15]
- Better physical health[16]
- More engagement in goal-directed planning[17]
- More resilience in response to change or failure[18]
- Lower all-cause death rate, including cardiovascular mortality[19]
- Better outcomes in the treatment of chronic diseases, including cancer[20]
- Less depression[21]
- Greater creativity and openness to new ideas[22]
- Better employee performance and organizational commitment and lower burnout and stress at work.[23]

So numerous are its positive associations that optimism has been called the "Velcro construct" because everything seems to stick to it.[24]

It could be that optimism causes benevolent outcomes or vice versa. Probably the influence flows in both directions in a virtuous cycle. Optimism is partly a self-fulfilling prophecy. For example, those who anticipate that other people will accept them tend to respond with interpersonal warmth, which increases the likelihood that others will in fact accept them.[25] Experiencing positive outcomes in turn reinforces optimism.[26]

Hazards of Optimism

There can be a darker side to optimism. High hopes can leave you vulnerable to disappointment, even danger. It is not always the case that the more optimistic you are, the better. Business and military disasters have been attributed to overconfidence.[27] Beyond the realities of unrealistic hope (Chapter 3), high optimism can create blind spots, particularly in underestimating risk. Optimistic people are more likely to regard themselves to be at less risk than others for bad things to happen to them.[28]

On a flight to Dallas I noticed that the bombastic fellow seated just in front of me didn't fasten his seatbelt when told to do so during the safety instructions. It hung down over the armrest into the aisle, and the busy flight attendants apparently didn't notice it. Should I point it out? (I didn't, although if he had been elderly I probably would have.) All through the flight he ignored the safety warnings to buckle up for takeoff, potential turbulence, and landing. I concluded that he must be an example of *it will never happen to me.*

I don't need to wear my bicycle helmet, Mom.

It's just too hot to work when I'm wearing all that protective gear.

I don't need to get a mammogram (or vaccine, or prostate exam); I feel fine.

I'm a really good driver, and I hate how the shoulder belt feels.

I don't need to wear sunscreen (or a condom, or a hat).

This is the *unrealistic optimism effect* in psychology: Most people believe that compared to others they are less susceptible to many adverse experiences, such as having an accident, or heart attack, or being the victim of a crime.[29]

High optimism is also associated with higher self-esteem and self-confidence, with a danger of explaining away negative outcomes rather than learning from them. Anything that might be regarded as a personal failure may be subjected to spin, attributing it to bad luck, other people's fault, or a temporary circumstantial exception to the usual pattern of success and competence.

Some folks, particularly pessimists, hold a cynical view of optimism. In Eleanor Porter's best-selling novel *Pollyanna*, the orphaned title character is uncommonly cheerful and optimistic despite hardship. In America at least, calling someone a Pollyanna is often meant to be sarcastically derogatory, denoting a foolishly hopeful person. Ironically to the contrary, Porter's Pollyanna, like the more recent stage and film orphan in *Annie*, benevolently transformed those around her to happy endings. Another undauntedly optimistic character is *Anne of Green Gables* in the novels by Lucy Maud Montgomery. Such optimism is also found in real life. Perhaps you have known someone with this kind of persistent cheerfulness. I have the good fortune of a few friends who consistently accentuate the positive. It has also been characteristic of our daughter Lillian, evident from the moment we first met her in the social worker's office. She has not only survived but flourished through daunting difficulties.[30] Optimistic people surely are not insulated from adversity or unhappiness, but optimism can help to carry them through hard times.

There seems to be a sweet spot in between too-high and too-low optimism.[31] In statistics it's called a curvilinear relationship, shaped like the McDonald's golden arch. It's not so good to be at either end, and the best place is in the middle. Students' test anxiety is like that. Very low physical arousal (perhaps through apathy, sleep deprivation, or a sedating drug) can lead to poor performance. Very high anxiety can interfere with effective test taking. In between is the Goldilocks level of just the right amount to facilitate attention, concentration, and a good test score. Optimism seems to be like that too.

Pessimism

So what about pessimism? A scale to measure pessimism contains items such as "If anything can possibly go wrong for me, it does," and "I hardly ever expect good things to happen." In some ways pessimism is the reverse of and a rejection of optimism. Just as optimists can explain away failures, it is equally possible for pessimists to dismiss achievements. Commenting on what she perceived to be an unmerited success, my skeptical great-grandmother would declare, "Even a blind hog finds an acorn once in a while."

And just as optimism is linked to a host of positive outcomes, pessimism as a personality characteristic is associated with poorer physical and emotional health.[32] A rare long-term study followed initially healthy and successful students at Harvard University. A pessimistic way of thinking at age 25 predicted physical illness as confirmed by physician examinations 20 to 35 years later, even after taking into account initial levels of physical and emotional health.[33]

However, optimism and pessimism are not directly opposite each other in the same way that warm and cold or tall and short are. They are more like masculinity and femininity, which were once regarded to be opposite characteristics such that if you were high on one you would automatically be low on the other. It turns out that it is possible to be androgynous—high in both masculine and feminine traits.[34] Similarly, a person who is high in optimism can have a pessimistic side. It is also possible to be neither optimistic nor pessimistic. Physical health is more closely related to the absence of pessimism than to the presence of optimism.[35] Said another way: In terms of health outcomes, pessimism is more bad news than optimism is good news, although both do matter.

As with optimism, pessimism has self-fulfilling properties. As mentioned in Chapter 2, those who expect social rejection are likely to behave cautiously or coldly toward others, thereby increasing the chances that they will be snubbed.[36] People with a strong external locus of control (Chapter 3) may have fatalistic beliefs that there is nothing they can do to change the future and therefore don't try—a pattern called *learned helplessness*.[37] Both animals and people can develop helplessness as a natural consequence of prolonged inability to escape painful experiences, which in turn can predispose to depression.[38] Individuals who already have an external locus of control more readily develop helplessness after failure experiences.[39] However, this fatalistic passivity and the related depression can be overcome or prevented by learning effective ways to exercise control over what can be changed.[40] Empowering experiences that strengthen a sense of personal control can foster *learned hopefulness*.[41] It may be a belief in one's personal ability that fosters such hopefulness, and it can also be a tribal hope for collective ability to achieve positive goals together.[42]

Pessimism can be a defensive mental strategy to protect self-esteem. If the expected outcome is always bad (pessimism), then failure is perfectly normal and any positive accomplishment is a pleasant surprise. This is not necessarily a problem. Low expectations can serve to lessen anxiety, making it more possible to try.[43] I am characteristically a hopeful person, but when administering complex organizations I have found it helpful to have a pessimistic colleague or two who anticipate anything and everything that could go wrong, a bit like a canary in a coal mine. I usually haven't succumbed to their gloom, but I have certainly paid attention to the potential pitfalls that they envisioned as a counterpoint to my preferred cheerful melody.

Contagion of Optimism and Pessimism

Optimism is infectious. You can pick it up, like a catchy tune, from others. Indeed, the concentration camp survivor Elie Wiesel remarked that hope can *only* be given to someone by other human beings.[44]

Fear, as you know, is likewise contagious. In a children's story, the chicken Henny Penny is knocked on the head by a dropping acorn and proceeds to spread lethal panic that "the sky is falling!" As in many churches nationwide, our congregation's membership has been decreasing and aging. One member spreads despair that "the church is dying!" The more optimistic, having seen congregations wax and wane over decades, perceive a new beginning. Either way, such visions can be self-perpetuating, like rumors of fuel shortages that prompt long gas station lines of cars with idling engines and can boost the sale of hybrid and electric vehicles. When viewing the same reality, people can embrace different conclusions that, if shared, will alter the reality for better or worse.

How do you become convinced of positive or negative expectations? Certainly the beliefs of those you care about matter. Opinions are more influential when they are expressed by people whom you regard to be similar to you in relevant ways.[45] More generally, people tend to make value judgments in relation to the views of one or more "reference groups" with which they identify and compare themselves, and that therefore can influence what they believe and value. A reference group might, for example, be members of a particular occupation, political party, or religious persuasion. You don't even have to be a member yourself to identify with a reference group; you may simply admire and aspire to be like them.[46] Reference groups vary in the amount of pressure exerted for uniformity among members.[47] Within several communities of which I am a member there are some clearly defined subgroups who share and reinforce each other's optimistic or pessimistic views regarding their collective future.

Who are the people in your reference groups whose opinions matter to you and who influence your own attitudes?

Sometimes discrete memorable experiences have a profound enduring effect on a person's outlook. In Dickens's *A Christmas Carol* the curmudgeonly Ebenezer Scrooge is transformed overnight to cheerfulness by an encounter with ghosts, as is Jimmy Stewart's character George Bailey by the unlikely angel Clarence in the classic film *It's a Wonderful Life*. Real people can be permanently changed for better or worse by sudden insights or epiphanies.[48] The enduring hopefulness of Julian of Norwich was planted by profound spiritual visions that she experienced while gravely ill.[49]

Both optimism and pessimism are mental biases with related brain systems.[50] As described in Chapter 2, these motivational biases influence what we notice and remember and also how we interpret what is happening. One such process is paying selective attention to positive or negative information that confirms our expectations. We begin looking for evidence and pay greater attention to what we hope for or fear. This process then strengthens the beliefs that prompted the search in the first place. When feeling fearful, we understandably scan the world for potential threats and become more anxious. Depressed people focus more on disheartening information, and angry people look for reasons to be outraged. Exposure to distressing pictures, stories, or news increases psychological distress, which further encourages vigilance for danger. For example, exposure to negative news media is associated with increased stress and anxiety as well as a felt urgency to continue checking, especially among pessimistic people.[51] People who are anxious or depressed generally spend more time being exposed to negative media that exacerbate their fear or pessimism.[52] What about *changes* in mental health? When bad news was omnipresent in several nations during the COVID-19 pandemic, the amount of time spent on the internet or watching television was associated with declines in mental health.[53]

In contrast, optimists pay more attention to hopeful information, right down to something as specific as how much time their eyes spend focusing on positive versus negative images.[54] This aspect of optimism could be problematic if it caused people to ignore important negative information (sometimes called "denial"). However, this does not appear to be the usual case. In fact, characteristically optimistic people actually tend to pay *more* attention to and know more about risk information, and on average they are healthier.

What can get you into trouble is *unrealistic* optimism—erroneously judging that your risk is lower than it actually is.[55] You might not want to go mountain climbing with a quixotically optimistic guide who believes that everything will be just fine. Unrealistic optimism is notorious in construction and development projects when estimating the amount of time and money that will be required. A classic example of mistaken optimism is tolerance for alcohol—being able to drink larger quantities than most people without feeling or appearing to be intoxicated. A common belief of high-tolerance people who can "hold their liquor" is that they are therefore at less risk from drinking than other people are. Just the opposite is true. Such tolerance can be measured sensitively by observing the extent to which a person's body sways at a particular dose of ethyl alcohol.[56] Such insensitivity or low response to alcohol is genetically influenced, and it is actually a significant risk factor for developing alcohol problems and related harm in both men and women: The greater the tolerance, the higher the risk.[57] It's rather like having no smoke alarm at home to warn you of danger.

Recognizing that optimism (like pessimism) loves company, "Optimist Clubs" began forming in the United States and Canada after World War I. A century later there are over 2,500 autonomous clubs worldwide focused on community service with particular emphasis on youth development. In a classic statement of optimism, the creed of Optimist International includes "to look at the sunny side of everything and make your optimism come true; to think only of the best, to work only for the best, and to expect only the best."[58]

Collective optimism or pessimism can shape the future. An example from economics is consumer confidence, which is used to anticipate sales, credit usage, and future economic conditions such as recession.[59] Collective optimism can rise or fall within a group or population, affecting people's willingness to invest in the future. Such future-oriented choices are as diverse as building up savings and investments, becoming pregnant, pursuing higher education, buying insurance, gifting endowments, and even taking steps to promote and protect your own health.[60] Effective leaders can foster a shared sense of collective agency, and people who are more hopeful as individuals more readily join in this shared optimism.[61]

Optimism can even affect the past. It colors how we remember and reinterpret what has already happened. History is often written by the victors and can have very different content when authored by the vanquished.[62] The phrase "sour grapes" originates from a story in Aesop's Fables in which a fox, after numerous unsuccessful attempts to reach a juicy bunch of grapes, concludes that they would have been sour anyway. It refers to the human tendency to devalue what we can't have. Similarly, it's just human nature to exaggerate one's own achievements and minimize shortcomings. The storyteller Garrison Keillor spun humorous tales of his fictional hometown Lake Wobegon, where "all the children are above average," lending its name to the *Lake Wobegon effect* in psychology in which most people regard themselves to be above average for various skills and abilities (such as safe driving) as well as below average in risk for a wide range of dangers—both of which obviously cannot be true. [63] This tendency is taken to extremes in narcissism, named for the mythic character Narcissus, who fell in love with his own reflection in a pool of water and spent the rest of his life staring at it. Narcissistic belief is that I am superior to others in intelligence, cleverness, and competence, that I ought to be widely admired, and that society would be perfect if only I could control it.

In sum, optimism is a personality characteristic that involves what you think, feel, and do about the future, with a general inclination to hope and expect that good things will occur.[64] As with hope more generally, optimism can be active—believing and acting as if your own efforts can make a difference in what happens—as well as passive: that good things will emerge (or bad things will be averted) through the efforts of others or through forces beyond your personal control. Though there are potential pitfalls, an optimistic style is overwhelmingly associated with a wide range of positive experiences and traits.

> How optimistic or pessimistic are you as a person? Do you think that your optimism is more active or passive?

As with desire, optimism is more likely to be impactful when accompanied by behavior that is consistent with a positive outlook. Collective action can be more effective than individual efforts alone. After receiving a heart transplant, a friend was advised by his health team to give his family and friends specific instructions. "Don't treat me with kid gloves, like I'm fragile or disabled. You can help me by relating to me like a normal person."

Beyond a characteristic style, optimism and pessimism are also ongoing in-the-moment choices of how to experience and respond to the present. You choose how to view every partially filled glass that you encounter, and an optimistic or pessimistic style is made up of one interpretation at a time over the course of time. When facing uncertainty, it matters what you choose because the benefit of the doubt is a benefit indeed in that perceptions shape the future.

Optimism can be donned like a garment. Indeed one choice at a time is how the attribute of optimism and its attendant benefits emerge.

In this chapter we have considered both active and passive facets of hoping. We turn now to a particular more passive form of hoping that nevertheless involves a choice: the decision of whether to trust.

TAKING IT PERSONALLY: OPTIMISM

- What kinds of experiences in your life may have inclined you to be more optimistic or pessimistic?

- In thinking of each of your parents or caregivers, would you say that they were more optimistic or pessimistic?

- Think of a person you know who is particularly pessimistic. How might their outlook have contributed to difficulties or unhappiness in the past or present?

CHAPTER 6

Trust

The best way to find out if you can trust somebody
is to trust them.

          —Ernest Hemingway

Have enough courage to trust love one more time
and always one more time.

          —Maya Angelou

Two graceful figures glide like pendulums high above
the center circus ring. Soaring on each trapeze, they syn-
chronize their swings, one hanging upside down with his
muscular arms outstretched, while the other grips the bar
and gains momentum, preparing for the trick. The precise moment arrives, and the flier releases just at the top
of her arc, tucking into a somersault before reaching out.
She does not merely wish for him to catch her. She knows
from long experience that he will. She trusts him.

Trust shares with other facets of hope the gem's core of anticipating
a benevolent future. Each aspect of hope is an angle from which
the future can be perceived. Probability is a calculation, possibility a vision, desire a wish, and optimism a predisposition. Trust is
more like a decision, a risky choice to entrust your well-being to the

safekeeping of another. It may be a momentary connection like a
rescue worker shouting "Take my hand!" or it can be the product
of long-shared experience. There is trust when you open your jaws
for the dentist or accept anesthesia before surgery. In a relationship
it is the opposite of fear: the mutual assurance of trapeze artists, of
seasoned police partners, and of lovers. Trust displaces fear.

In some ways trust is like optimism, but it is attached to particular people or objects. You confide in certain people more than others and trust your bicycle or vehicle to get you to your destination.
Some situations you trust, while others you fear. Such confidence is
usually based on prior experience with the person or situation, and
thereby, unlike optimism, it is earned.

I remember clearly the moment when our younger boy, Jay-
son, took his first hesitant jump into our waiting arms in a swimming pool. Soon he was climbing out and repeating the leap with
glee: "Again, again!" It was all the more deeply moving in light of
his traumatic start in life before moving in with us at 15 months
of age. During the first week after he came to us, as I held him in
my arms against my chest, he would twist around anxiously as if
struggling to see what was going on behind him. Gradually over a
few more weeks he settled in, snuggled, and relaxed as we held him.
However, he showed no distress if we stepped out of the room, from
which fact our family therapist concluded that he must have been
left alone often. So much had already happened before he even had
any language to understand or describe it!

The psychologist Erik Erikson posited eight stages of human
development that build on each other from infancy through old
age.[1] Each answers a basic existential question, the first of which is
whether the world is a safe and trustworthy place. Should I trust or
mistrust the world and people around me? If I cry, is anyone going

to come? Will somebody be there for me? People normally resolve this question one way or the other within the first 18 months of life, so we took our boy home quite late in this stage of growth. With reliable, loving care children can develop a basic sense of trust and security to carry them through future situations and relationships, a durable hope that can sustain them even through hardships and adversity. On the other hand, if this first stage of development resolves instead toward hopelessness, there can be an enduring propensity to be mistrustful, anxious, and angry.

In the course of living it is possible to have *corrective emotional experiences* that challenge prior assumptions and predispositions.[2] They can occur in psychotherapy and also within healthy nurturing relationships. Establishing trust is an important first step in many helping professions.[3] Someone who by virtue of their life experience generally expects to be treated in an adverse way (criticized, judged, or punished, for example) may find a welcome and healing exception in a trusted therapist, friend, or caregiver.

Animals too can trust or mistrust. Horses evolved as flight animals, well equipped to be wary of and to outrun potential predators. A traditional way of convincing horses to obey was to "break" them through weeks of domination and violence. (This is also, by the way, a now discredited method for treating addiction—to "break them down to build them up."[4]) The original horse whisperer, Monty Roberts, developed a learnable, nonviolent method for "joining up" that within skillful hands can invite an untamed horse to accept its first blanket, saddle, and rider within half an hour without inflicting pain.[5] If a horse has already been physically abused, join-up can take much longer. I watched Monty working successfully with one such horse that was so dangerous it would have been killed had his method failed.[6] On its flanks it bore the marks of a chain with which it had been whipped. More recently Monty has been teaching his join-up method to military veterans suffering from combat-induced post-traumatic stress injury in which learning to trust is a formidable challenge.[7]

Join-up involves two-way trust. I had the privilege of experiencing it myself alone in a round pen with a horse I had never met while Monty coached me from the observation railing. For a few minutes the filly fled around the perimeter first in one direction, then in the other as I followed with my eyes and posture. *No getting away from this strange man!* As instructed, I watched the galloping horse for specific signals of willingness to have a "conversation" with me: slightly slowing pace, drifting a bit sideways toward me, dropping her head with some chewing motions. Then at a precise moment as directed, I turned my back on the horse and slowly walked into the center of the ring, where I stopped. I could hear that she had stopped too, and I waited. "Now look over your shoulder," Monty said. I did, and there at my back was the horse's nose, waiting as if to say, "OK, now what?" This moment of join-up is just the beginning of developing trust. As you can imagine, turning your back on a thousand-pound animal is a courageously difficult act of trust for traumatized soldiers when learning this method.[8]

We also place our trust in inanimate objects like a rope, a ladder, or a satellite navigation system. Stepping into an elevator involves a certain amount of trust, perhaps with some reassurance from a posted certificate of inspection. Most people enter an elevator without giving it much thought, although some suffer intense fear. A classic psychology experiment was designed to determine when infants develop depth perception. A baby would crawl toward the mother across a clear glass sheet that at first had a solid checkerboard surface beneath it, but then came to a *visual cliff* where the floor seemed to drop away, giving the appearance of open space. Once depth perception has developed, most babies will stop short at the apparent drop-off even though they could continue crawling safely. Such fear has obvious survival value. There are modern entertainment versions of the visual cliff at tall buildings, towers, and the Grand Canyon that offer clear platforms allowing brave folks to walk out over a sheer drop where their depth perception battles mightily against the hopeful trust that the transparent floor is dependable.

As a boy scout I learned and trusted the stars, using the constellations to know where I was going. Twenty-five years later in Australia when I looked up at the night sky I recognized nothing at all. It's hard to describe what a deeply disturbing feeling I had to see nothing where it was supposed to be.

When one is faced with risk and uncertainty, a physical object like a child's blanket may instill comfort. Some people experience security from the presence of a religious object or a trusted companion. Uniforms can instill trust, wariness, or fear depending on one's prior experience. An insignia or flag may be idolized, imbued with ultimate reverence and trust, as can a person, an organization, a cause, even an idea or ideology.[9] The hope is that you are not alone but are accompanied by what is reliable and dependable.

Predisposition to Trust

One of many ways in which we differ as people is in our tendency to trust or mistrust. As mentioned earlier, this general inclination develops quite early in life. At one end the tendency is to distrust everyone unless and until they demonstrate

> Where do you fall on this predisposition from broad trust to general mistrust?

themselves to be trustworthy. "Prove that I can trust you" is a difficult challenge. Trust can be hard to earn and easy to lose, particularly for people at this guarded end of the spectrum. At the opposite extreme are those who trust as their default assumption unless someone shows that they do not deserve it, and even well beyond that point. In between are varying degrees of cautiousness.

Beyond a general willingness to give people the benefit of the doubt, your inclination to trust may vary depending on someone's appearance and mannerisms even at first impression. Unusual appearance or behavior can make people wary. Skin color, dress, or idiosyncrasies like shifting eyes may affect others' ease or unease. Newly hired employees often have a formal or informal probation period during which their honesty and reliability are observed, and employers differ in how readily they form these impressions. Within a society, skilled occupations vary in their perceived trustworthiness. What is your own predisposition to trust doctors, airline pilots, therapists, lawyers, or clergy? In ancient Israel, shepherds fell at the very bottom in respect and trustworthiness, making it all the more shocking that in Luke's gospel they were the only ones invited to witness a holy arrival.[10]

Earned or not, being trusted is a privilege. In both the financial and prison systems, trustees are those invested with special responsibility. What is it that inspires trust, whether in business or personal relationships? Trust is gained by being honest and respectful and by meeting expectations. A starting point in trustworthiness then is understanding what is expected of you. As an employer I generally wanted our work to be done well and on time, with some allowance for learning new tasks, human fallibility, and life's unexpected intrusions. My responsibility was to communicate clearly what I expected and when. I had the good fortune of hiring two remarkable women who worked with me as administrators for 20 years and contributed mightily to what we were able to accomplish during that time. They had to train me in how to work with them, with the essence being "trust us and let us do our job." I soon learned that they would do what was needed early and well without my needing to hover or double-check. What a privilege! In personal and intimate relationships there is a similar challenge of understanding each other's hopes, desires, and expectations and not violating trust.

There is mutual vulnerability in a two-way relationship of trust. Effective counselors are trustworthy in professional conduct, such as confidentiality, and are also willing to share something of themselves when there is good reason to believe that it will benefit their clients. It is also important for professional helpers to trust the wisdom and resources of those whom they serve, honoring their freedom to make their own choices. Mutual trust is closely related to happiness in personal relationships, organizations, and nations.[11] Personal acts of kindness, such as "paying it forward" and volunteering with charitable organizations, seem to strengthen this link.[12] Contributing to others' well-being can enhance your own sense of trust and happiness. Being reliable and responsible promotes trust.

Placing high personal or cultural value on independence may reflect a reluctance to trust others. A psychiatrist from India, Salvador Neki, was puzzled by what seemed to him to be a loathing of dependence in Western cultures. People, he observed, seem pressured to become independent as soon as possible, and then if they ever have to depend on others again, it's considered shameful. In India, he said, children are encouraged to enjoy their childhood and then move from dependence to being *dependable*.[13] Later in life it is normal to rely on others again. If society has only dependent and independent people, Dr. Neki asked, then who is dependable?

It is so easy to focus on problems: what's wrong, what's not going well. In contrast, the field of positive psychology is the study of what contributes to human potential, to happiness, hope, and success.[14] The method of *appreciative inquiry*, for example, seeks to discover, explore, and build on positive strengths.[15] What is *best* about, what gives life and joy to this individual, group, or organization? What is going well; what are you proud of? What might be possible and how could it happen? Such positive questions can call out the best in a person or group and can contribute to building a culture of mutual trust and hope.[16]

What happens when hope has been vested in trusting someone or something, and then the trust is violated? Like a decision, trust can also change in a moment, sometimes too late, as in the famous line "Et tu, Brute?" (You, too, Brutus?) in Shakespeare's *Julius Caesar*, when the emperor suddenly recognizes a close friend among his assassins.[17] Violation of trust, though usually nonlethal, can change someone's faith in a person if not in humanity more generally, and recovering a willingness to trust again can be terribly difficult. Such was the story of a teenage boy who fled his violent father to enter a monastery, only to be sexually abused years later by his priest confessor there. His healing took place over a period of 20 years, and the story ends well with James Finley becoming both a psychotherapist and a spiritual mentor who has helped countless others, including me.[18]

Your Role in Trusting

Trust could be understood as passive, meaning that the hope (and therefore the responsibility) for betterment is vested in forces beyond yourself. In classic western films, the helpless and beleaguered townspeople tell their savior–hero that "You are our only hope." Yet trust in others or institutions need not preclude, and indeed can inspire, your own active involvement. In health care you can sit back and depend on your doctors to do the work or you can take a personal role and responsibility for your own health. Particularly in managing long-term health challenges, what you choose to do or not do in daily life has a major influence on your future wellness and quality of life. Beyond your own proclivity for optimism (Chapter 5) at least three other factors contribute to your trusting: evidence, emotion, and grace.

One consideration then is whether trust is warranted given the *evidence,* including past experience. Is this person or product reliable? Prior behavior or performance creates expectations for trustworthiness, whether it's about a person, an organization, or a maker of automobiles.[19] Hucksters sell hope in products that have little or no evidence of benefit beyond the placebo effect discussed in Chapter 4. Erich Fromm distinguished rational faith, grounded in proven reliability and trustworthiness, from irrational faith, "which one accepts as true regardless of whether it is or not."[20] Although the implication here is that there are only two kinds of hope or trust—rational and irrational—there are many gradations in between rational and irrational hope. As demonstrated by the use of courtroom juries, evidence is partly in the eye of the beholder. How trustworthy is this source or person? How strong and reliable is the evidence? Is there a reasonable doubt? Even scientific evidence is often stated as a probability (Chapter 3).[21] One contribution that you make to trust then is in choosing what sources and evidence you accept as sufficient or convincing.

Beyond rationality, there are important *emotional* components of trust and mistrust. In considering whether to trust, part of the equation is how we *feel* about the person or object. Our own current emotional state, whether positive or negative, affects our willingness to trust. We are more likely to trust when feeling happy and to mistrust when we're angry or anxious.[22] Consider the issue of trusting artificial intelligence, such as a self-driving vehicle. People who were already feeling anxious before taking a simulated test drive were less trusting of the automation.[23] Judgments about someone's trustworthiness are also influenced by the person's own expressed emotions. We are more likely to trust people who appear to be happy or grateful than those expressing a negative emotion like anger.[24] There's a reason salespeople put on a happy face.

The act of trusting can in itself invoke a feeling of comfort and safety, although fear can overwhelm it. Trustworthiness involves thinking and judgment, whereas fear is a primitive survival emotion that is rooted in a much older part of the brain. In the *Dune* novels, Frank Herbert described fear as "the mind killer," linked to fight, flight, or freeze. It can override thinking and judgment, favoring rigid beliefs over flexibility, caution instead of creativity, aggression rather than cooperation.[25] Emotional predisposition can narrow selective attention, shaping how we view reality. Fear favors vigilance, mistrust, and avoidance rather than curiosity, openness, and attraction.

It is also possible to grant unearned trust, sometimes known as *grace*. A person's capacity to trust others can be inspired by the experience of *being* trusted, even if it was the undeserved variety. Early in Victor Hugo's novel *Les Misérables,* the kindly Bishop Myriel admits a stranger, the recently released convict Jean Valjean, into his home, offering him supper and a place to sleep. During the night Valjean slips out with stolen silverware, and when apprehended he lies that the bishop gave it to him. The police escort him back to the scene of the crime, where the bishop sets the foundation for the rest of the novel by confirming Valjean's untrue story and further giving him two precious silver candlesticks that he had "forgotten" to take with him, reminding Valjean that he had promised to become an honest man. The bishop's unmerited trust ultimately inspires a permanent life change.

Like forgiveness, trust is a decision that only you can make. You can choose to trust despite doubts and fear. If the risk is rewarded, trusting can open the door to further trust just as fear begets more fear. As conveyed in *Les Misérables*, offering someone unjustified trust may inspire trustworthiness, and at least affords an opportunity to demonstrate it. How many times should we forgive or trust? "As many as seven times?" a disciple asked the wisdom teacher. "Not seven, but seventy-seven times" was the rabbi's startling answer—in other words, beyond our ability to keep count.[26] Grace is extending trust beyond what someone deserves.

> Think about the people you have trusted most. How do you decide whether someone is a person you should trust?

Trusting Yourself

Trust and grace can be extended not only to others but to yourself as well. Self-confidence can be a particular challenge for some, though we generally tend to be differentially charitable toward ourselves. This is a well-documented psychological finding called the *better-than-average effect* (or the Lake Wobegon effect from Chapter 5), particularly found for desirable skills and traits such as fairness, fitness, listening ability, and intelligence.[27] We may even compare ourselves favorably to others in humility.[28] A large majority of motor vehicle operators say that they are above-average drivers. In one study, 94 percent of college professors rated themselves as above-average teachers, and two-thirds ranked themselves in the top 25 percent.[29]

Some obvious hazards of overconfidence are complacency (for example, failing to study for a test) and lack of inclination to improve. Ironically it is the most skillful people who tend to underestimate their ability, whereas those with lower ability seem to be quite unaware of it ("I've got this! No problem!").[30] Unlike surgeons, psychotherapists rarely become more skillful with years of practice.[31] The most effective therapists are those who devote additional deliberate time and effort to practice and keep on developing their skills beyond the hours spent with their clients, just as musicians devote many hours to practicing apart from performances.[32] Perhaps humility regarding your own expertise motivates continuous effort to improve, thereby yielding greater skill.

I had quite a humbling experience in this regard when I decided to evaluate my own teaching. As a university professor I had already received myriad subjective ratings from students, but my specific interest on this occasion was in how well people were actually learning the skill that I wanted to teach them. The proficiency to be learned was the clinical skill of motivational interviewing, and the trainees were professional probation counselors.[33] Immediately following a 2-day clinical workshop and then again 4 months later we asked for the usual written evaluations of the training, how much they had learned, and the extent to which they were using the training in their day-to-day work. This time though we also recorded audio samples of the trainees' counseling sessions with supervisees before and after the workshop, and had trained observers code the recordings for specific component skills that had been covered during the workshop.[34] On participants' self-report ratings we received glowing reviews for the quality of the training, their increased proficiency with motivational interviewing, and how useful they found their newly acquired skills to be in their daily work. Actual practice behavior, however, had changed very little. There was no decrease in counselors' talk time, questions, or responses inconsistent with motivational interviewing and no change in how their clients were responding. Four months after the training there was very little evidence that I had been there. What I had inspired was false confidence.

It stung, of course, but I should not have been surprised. Closely related to the better-than-average effect is the *Dunning–Kruger effect,* which, rudely stated, is that we are blissfully unaware of our inability, and it is the lowest performers who most overestimate their competence.[35] I could have blamed the students for not learning, but the responsibility was mine. Clearly I had not effectively taught what I wanted them to learn. The study did help us ask better questions. Instead of "Did it work?" we began asking "What does it take to learn this complex skill?" We soon found that a modest amount of additional feedback and coaching based on observed practice was enough to help trainees learn and retain proficiency in clinical skills.[36]

It is possible though difficult to judge our own ability accurately. On rating scales like "How good a listener are you?" we tend to be inaccurate judges of our own skillfulness or, said another way, our self-ratings don't correspond well to ratings from objective observers. It is more possible to accurately count specific responses in recordings of your own work: How many times did you do specific things, such as ask a question, practice reflective listening, or offer encouragement? I still remember the first time I watched (along with graduate student peers and a professor) a videotape of myself as an interviewer. I was embarrassed and seriously considered going into another line of work, but that's a common experience when first observing yourself in practice. I now know that reviewing recordings is one of the most valuable forms of intentional practice to improve interpersonal skills, ideally in the company of a supportive coach and peers. It's often used in helping people learn skills in sports, music, or public speaking.

"Trust, but verify" is a rhyming Russian proverb (*doveryai, no proveryai*) that President Ronald Reagan introduced in international negotiations on nuclear disarmament. *Trust but verify* can be particularly wise when appraising ourselves. In the absence of verifying information we are prone to overestimate our own abilities and virtues, thereby undermining motivation to improve. Being observed while learning new skills is common and an essential element of training in many fields, such as music, medicine, and acting. In sports like tennis and golf, when we ask someone with expertise to coach us, we would never say, "But don't watch me—I'd be too embarrassed." Asking for observation and guidance is an act of trust, both in a teacher or mentor and in yourself.

As a form of hope, trust places confidence in a particular person or object. It is different from betting on statistical probability, possibility, desire, or general optimism. It's not necessarily based on past experience. Someone requesting help from a professional (such as a plumber, doctor, technician, or advisor) may have had no prior exposure to that person and will likely be paying close attention to judge their trustworthiness, rather like test-driving a vehicle before purchasing it. Trust is a choice and a relationship of hope.

Whereas trust is often external, vested in someone or something beyond yourself, other forms of hope seem to focus more on internal experience. The next chapter considers how hope can arise from the meaning and purpose we find in what happens.

TAKING IT PERSONALLY: TRUST

- When have you had good results from choosing to be vulnerable and trust someone?

- Can you think of a "corrective emotional experience" from your own life or that of someone you know?

- When do you think that "trust and verify" is appropriate, and when is it better just to trust someone?

- When has someone extended grace—unearned trust or forgiveness—to you?

CHAPTER 7

Meaning and Purpose

Hope is not a feeling of certainty that everything
ends well. Hope is just a feeling that life and work
have a *meaning* . . . the certainty that something
makes sense, regardless of how it turns out.

—Vaclav Havel

We are not called to be successful, but to be
faithful.

—Mother Teresa

Having landed a role that would soon make him famous,
the 6'4" Christopher Reeve bulked up his slender body to
fill out his suit, so much so that some of the earliest-shot
scenes of the first Superman movie had to be refilmed
because his appearance had changed so dramatically.
The film was a huge success, and he soared through two
sequels.

Then, at 42, Reeve was riding in an equestrian com-
petition when his horse stopped abruptly just before a
jump, catapulting him across the fence. He landed hard,
and the top two vertebrae of his spine were crushed, leaving him paralyzed from the neck down.[1]

His unprecedented hope was to walk again before
turning 50. Though medical experts discouraged this

goal, he tried a variety of treatments and did manage to regain some sensation and movement, becoming an intrepid public advocate for finding a way to cure paralysis. He died at 52, and the Christopher & Dana Reeve Foundation continues his search by funding research on spinal cord injury and its treatment.

Why are we here? As far as we know, it's not a question that other creatures ask themselves, but at least some humans do. Some people wander the world in search of meaning and purpose in life. Friedrich Nietzsche observed that someone "who has a why to live for can bear almost any how." Optimism is a penchant for anticipating positive endings across many spheres of life, while trust finds a specific source of confidence. We turn now to yet a different facet of hope: finding meaning or purpose in whatever is happening, whether benevolent or not.

Meaning in Life

Meaning and purpose are different, though related. Perceiving *meaning* in life can provide a sense of coherence, recognition, and comprehension in whatever is happening. It might, for example, be perceived as the gradual working out of a grand design, such as the socioeconomic theory of Karl Marx, a hidden organized conspiracy, or the spiritual progression of a cosmic plan. Meaning can be perceived from afar without having an individual part in or responsibility for it. *Purpose* in life includes a personal role in the present and future.

In 1952, as yet another brutal war began just a few years after World War II, a team of writers was commissioned to compose a song for a TV show to offer the public some hope. The song that they wrote, "I Believe," was the first hit song ever introduced on TV, and it became widely popular in the United States and particularly in the United Kingdom, where it set a still-unbroken record with 35 consecutive weeks in the top-10 singles chart. Its lyrics conveyed hopeful meaning in and beyond present difficulties. It was recorded by dozens of popular artists, including Frankie Laine, Louis Armstrong, Elvis Presley, and Barbra Streisand, and has been performed by countless choirs and choruses. There seems to be a human hunger to find meaning in life.

Meaning draws on your deeply held beliefs and values, painting a larger picture than the particulars of the present.[2] It provides a larger context within which to understand current adversity, a bit like zooming up to a certain altitude that affords a broader view. A sense of meaning in and beyond what is happening can offer some distance from current difficulties.[3] For oppressed people, a vision of future freedom, even if remote, can be a source of hope. Such hope is found in African American spirituals that emerged during the travail of slavery, where the words *home, Canaan,* and *promised land* could anticipate actual freedom in this life. Some songs like "Follow the Drinking Gourd" contained coded directions for a path to freedom, the "gourd" referring to the constellation Ursa Major or the Big Dipper that in the Northern Hemisphere points toward the North Star.

Meaning-hope can be a confident vision that there is a better future toward which history is moving inexorably, even if not quickly or steadily. Such hopeful inevitability was conveyed in the final "mountaintop" speech of Dr. Martin Luther King Jr. on the evening before he was assassinated:

Like anybody, I would like to live a long life. Longevity has its
place. But I'm not concerned about that now. I just want to do
God's will. And He's allowed me to go up to the mountain.
And I've looked over. And I've seen the promised land. I may
not get there with you. But I want you to know tonight, that
we, as a people, will get to the promised land.[4]

Mahatma Gandhi similarly trusted that the "truth force"
(*Satyāvgraha*) of nonviolent resistance would ultimately overcome
oppression, and his individual vision became a social movement.
Inevitability hope is the Shakespearean confidence that in the end
"the truth will out" and what is hidden will ultimately come to
light. As I write, the people of Ukraine manifest a collective resolve
to outlast the invasion of their nation.

Some forms of meaning-hope *transcend* material reality. Certain world religions, for example, offer promise of a better future
in reincarnation or an afterlife free from suffering.[5] Twelve-step
recovery programs like Alcoholics Anonymous, which are sometimes misunderstood as "self-help" groups, instead place faith in a
Higher Power: "We came to believe that a Power greater than ourselves could restore us to sanity."[6]

Hope is about possible futures, whether clearly envisioned or
simply trusted. Sometimes a lack of hope is an inability to imagine any future different from the present. "It's all I've ever known,"
someone might say truthfully of a life that has been dominated by
violence, abuse, drugs, and poverty. An envisioned future can be
shattered suddenly when events such as a stroke, imprisonment, or a
hurricane intervene, and it can be stressful even to hope for a better
future, let alone make plans for it.[7] When a loved one has suddenly
disappeared and their status is unknown, the loss is ambiguous and

possible futures can dissolve.[8] Having survived Nazi concentration camps, the psychiatrist Viktor Frankl developed a new form of psychotherapy called *logotherapy* to help people discover or recover meaning in their lives.[9]

Apart from specific imaginings of the future, one may have faith in the meaningfulness of life, even if the meaning is elusive. This is a conviction that there must be significance in suffering or tragedy.[10] An opposite view is nihilism: that there is no inherent or hidden meaning in life, and thus if you are going to have meaning you must create your own.[11] Either way, meaning matters.

Quantum Change

One's sense of meaning in life can be changed dramatically by sudden insights or epiphanies, as in the story of Ebenezer Scrooge in the 1843 Charles Dickens tale, *A Christmas Carol.* In 1902 William James called this the "self-surrender type" of change, describing abrupt and enduring transformations that are unlike the more familiar experience of gradual changes with two steps forward and one step back. Does this actually happen in real life?

Having personally studied this phenomenon, I am clear that it does occur and that such human metamorphoses are not rare.[12] Those who have had such a *quantum change* remember the experience vividly even decades later. Our research group interviewed 55 such people who were eager to tell us their story and were fascinated to learn that others had had such experiences. It is a distinctive, out-of-the-ordinary event that typically spans a few minutes or hours, a strange enough experience that most people had told no one or very few about what had happened. It took them by surprise, and they had a clear sense that they were not doing this themselves.

The changes that occurred were profoundly benevolent and seemingly permanent, as if they had passed through a one-way door. When interviewed about their experiences again 10 years later, they reported that their transformation had endured and often expanded.[13]

In a way, what had changed for them was their sense of meaning or purpose in life. Such changes sometimes occur with near-death experiences,[14] though none of those whom we interviewed had been close to death when it happened. About half had been in severe stress or pain, whereas many others were, like Scrooge, simply going about their ordinary lives when the unexpected arrived. Often their values were upended; what had formerly been most important now took a back seat, and previously less-prized aspects became central. Men and women each moved away from sex-role stereotypes and became more like each other. They impressed us as deeply peaceful, secure, and hopeful people. Many of them asked, "Why me? How was I, of all people, so fortunate to have had this experience?"

There are also darker transformations when life is abruptly turned upside down, as when suffering the death of a child, losing a job and career, or being a victim of violence. Such was Christopher Reeve's sudden injury and paralysis. One's familiar routines and sacred assumptions in life are upended. It can feel like being shattered or lost at sea, like all the pieces of one's life are suddenly cast up in the air and scattered to the winds. They may become

> When in your own life so far have your experienced a crisis or psychological struggle that eventually resulted in positive growth?

spiritual or existential struggles: Who am I now? How am I going to live? Why am I here? What's the point? As distressing as they are, these crises can also result in growth and new life.[15] In fact, Erik Erikson's theory of development (mentioned in Chapter 6) is that growth emerges from responding to the psychological crises of successive stages of life.

Hopeful Living

There are some broad hopeful perspectives on meaning in life. One of them is living with an outlook of gratitude, appreciating even small things. This mindset actively resists feeling entitled or taking kindness and pleasures for granted. It can be felt in simple acts like slowing down to enjoy birdsong or a sunset. Gratitude includes noticing, savoring, and acknowledging what is good even in the midst of adversity. Such perspectives can become part of a culture. In Costa Rica, the phrase *pura vida* conveys a sense of gratitude for what one does have in life. Like *aloha* in Hawaiian, *pura vida* can be a gracious form of greeting or farewell and also a way of life. When misfortune befalls—a canceled flight, a missed opportunity— saying *pura vida* is a way of slowing down and keeping things in larger perspective. Once in Pennsylvania while visiting an Amish community I asked a fellow why they shun automobiles in favor of horse and buggy, and his reply surprised me. "Automobiles give you hurry-up disease," he said. The Swahili phrase *hakuna matata* that was popularized in the play and film *The Lion King* advocates living simply and appreciating the beauty of life. In Norwegian and Danish, the cultural value of *hygge* conveys cozy togetherness as well as a psychological state of contentment and wholeness.[16]

Hope can also manifest as an existential commitment to life's journey without attachment to particular outcomes, a trustful contentment to live without closure.[17] In the words of the French priest and scientist Pierre Teilhard de Chardin, whose books were banned by the Catholic Church during his lifetime, "I am content to walk right to the end along a road of which I am more and more certain, toward an horizon more and more shrouded in mist."[18]

Purpose in Life

Having *purpose* includes perceived meaning in life as well as a meaningful personal role to perform with implications for *how* to live. Our purpose in life (PIL) is what we are *for*, what we are here for, not merely what we are against or fear.[19] It often is reflected in devotion to a person, organization, cause, or duty. Like optimism, having purpose in life (PIL) predicts longevity, life satisfaction, psychological well-being, and healthy aging,[20] whereas lower PIL is linked to anxiety, demoralization, depression, and medical illness.[21] For people with substance use disorders, demoralization is linked with a greater risk of relapse.[22] Meaning and purpose in life are particularly important issues for senior citizens, because a sense of PIL normally tends to diminish with aging.[23] Besides its broader links with physical and mental health across the lifespan, PIL is associated with significantly decreased risk of dementia with aging.[24] One possible contributing factor is that seniors with higher PIL are more likely to keep up-to-date with preventive health screening and services and to spend fewer nights in the hospital.[25] Experiencing PIL is linked to social integration (vs. isolation) and the number and quality of social relationships.[26] A couple in their 80s once offered me sage advice on aging: "Make younger friends."

PIL is also an important resource when coping with chronic illness.[27] Our research group offered psychological consultation

> If you were to write a "mission statement" describing the purpose of your life, what would it be?

for New Heart, a 12-week cardiovascular rehabilitation program in Albuquerque providing dietary and exercise coaching for people who had recently suffered a heart attack.[28] Our focus was on finding patients' own motivations to make the needed long-term lifestyle changes. Initially we assumed that not having another heart attack would be a prime sufficient motivator, but as it turned out a key question was "What do you have to live for?" Fear of dying proved to be a less potent impetus for change than their own reasons for longevity.

> I want to meet my grandchildren.
>
> I still have important work to do.
>
> My family needs me.
>
> It's time for me to start enjoying life.

These were the inner voices that helped people start or keep on exercising, decrease life stressors, and change their eating habits. They had a reason to live.

Prophetic Hope

Prophecy is concerned with the future and therefore overlaps with the domain of hope. Not primarily about predicting coming events, prophets envision a better future and impatiently offer a meaning-filled critique of the present along with prescriptive advice for how to live.[29] They see how we could and should be. The futures envisioned by Mahatma Gandhi and Dr. King called people to a purpose in life, a nonviolent way of living that would realize the vision.

Foreseeing what will or may come to pass, prophets offer hope as well as criticism of the present, often impelled to say and do disturbing things that run completely counter to the popular politics of their time. None of the biblical Hebrew prophets were delighted with their calling or message. In Jeremiah's case, for 20 years he had been preaching the downfall of his own nation, a doom that would ultimately fall upon himself as well. As you can imagine, this prophecy did not make him popular. Terrorized by the prospect of their country being invaded, the people of Judea clung to visions of national glory and assurances that God was on their side and would protect them. To the kings of Judea, Jeremiah counseled negotiation and submission to the enemy. It's no surprise then that, like many ancient and modern prophets, he suffered ostracism, imprisonment, and attempts on his life. And then it happened.

Travel back to the sixth century B.C.E., a dark turning point in the life of the kingdom of Judea and its capital, Jerusalem. The kingdom found itself between two powerful warring empires: Assyria and Egypt. The nationalistic King Josiah, who had formed an alliance with Babylon, was captured and executed by the Egyptians. His son Jehoiakim then placed his bets on Egypt and stopped paying tribute to Babylon. As a result, the Assyrian king, Nebuchadnezzar, invaded Jerusalem and exiled the royalty, the educated, the leaders, priests, and prophets to Babylon, near modern Baghdad.

Imagine it. The city you have lived in all your life is conquered by a neighboring superpower. Many of your friends and neighbors are dead, along with some of your family. Your name appears on a list of suspects, and one night, soldiers knock on your door, arrest you, and transport you to a far-off land as a prisoner. You don't speak the language. You don't like the food. You despise the national religion. Everything that is familiar to you—your community, home, schools, places of worship, work, loved ones, wealth—is gone. As a hated foreigner you will always have only menial drudge work, no influence, and you will live in poverty until the day you die.

That is the forlorn group to whom Jeremiah addressed a letter. He was left behind in Jerusalem because he had been publicly advocating submission to Babylon and was therefore regarded as a loyal friend of the occupying army. So what does Jeremiah now say to his people in exile, living in Babylon? Rather than "I told you so," he offers these words of advice, imagining a hopeful future in their present circumstances:

> Build houses and live in them; plant gardens and eat what they produce. Take wives and have sons and daughters; take wives for your sons, and give your daughters in marriage, that they may bear sons and daughters; multiply there, and do not decrease. But seek the welfare of the city where I have sent you into exile, and pray to the Lord on its behalf, for in its welfare you will find your welfare.[30]

Seeing meaning in what was happening, he counseled acting with hope and living with purpose. Some years later, Jeremiah would have the opportunity to follow his own advice. Jerusalem had once again rebelled against Babylon, and King Nebuchadnezzar once more besieged the city, cutting off its supplies. Death roamed the streets, and this time starvation was so severe that the people had resorted to cannibalism. The Assyrian army was literally at the gates and within a few days would breach the wall, slaughter its inhabitants, and burn the city to the ground. It was on this day that Jeremiah received news of the death of his cousin, which by law gave him first rights to purchase a field that the cousin owned. It was not exactly a seller's market, but Jeremiah assembled the required witnesses and purchased the field as a prophetic act of hope.

Eighteen hundred years later, a young Italian priest also lived in a time of widespread fear of a terrifying enemy. The year was 1219, and Europe's adversaries were the nations of Islam, vilified as an evil empire. The crusades had already been a military disaster for 120 years, destroying Middle Eastern cities and countless lives on both sides. With the blessing of the Church, the armies of the fifth crusade had marched off to attack Egypt once again, trying to reclaim the holy lands. In this fearful time, when any talk of negotiation suggested weakness, the young priest struggled with his conscience. If he spoke his mind and heart, he would surely be considered a fool and a traitor, perhaps even excommunicated. If he kept silent, he knew that he could never live with his own conscience. So he traveled to the front, to Egypt, to meet with both Islamic and Christian leaders, to counsel peace and mutual understanding. He failed, as did the fifth, sixth, seventh, and eighth crusades over the next 50 years. He was unsuccessful in stopping the war, but he had been true to his conscience and purpose in life, doing what little he could to promote peace and hope. His name was Francis of Assisi.

Seven hundred years later, a young Jew named Elie Wiesel would be among the survivors of the Nazi death camps, where millions were slaughtered. For the next 50 years of his life, Wiesel would struggle with his traumatized loss of faith and with how one can live in a world where such monstrous evil is possible. In his biography, *Elie Wiesel: Messenger to All Humanity*, Robert McAfee Brown recounted the stages of darkness through which Wiesel passed, as reflected in his writings. Is the world a hopelessly evil place? Should one withdraw into despair? Finally, after decades of spiritual struggle, Wiesel resolved that with or without God, the way to live with integrity in a world possessed by evil is to live *against* that evil, to commit whatever time and resources you have to make a positive difference.

Like the ancient and modern prophets, it is possible to experience hope and despair together. It is not necessary to choose between them, for both contain truth and hold possibilities for the future.[31] Elie Wiesel, Dr. King, and Mahatma Gandhi all faced head-on the reality of their times, as did Dolores Huerta in cofounding the United Farm Workers; Fannie Lou Hamer, who rose from poverty in Mississippi to become a leading voice in the civil and voting rights movements; and Sunitha Krishnan, who founded Prajwala in India, which rescues and rehabilitates victims of sex trafficking. They all grieved the stunning violence and oppression suffered by their people and refused to do nothing about it. Hope and distress share the crucible of the future and together can fuel perseverance.

TAKING IT PERSONALLY: MEANING AND PURPOSE

- How is it possible to hope and despair simultaneously? Is that experience familiar to you?

- If meaning is a framework through which you experience and make sense of life, what is the frame through which you currently view what happens to and around you? How did you come to have that perspective on life?

- Have you or someone you know had an experience that suddenly and dramatically changed the sense of meaning and purpose in life? How did it happen?

CHAPTER 8

Perseverance

Fall down seven times, stand up eight.
—Japanese Proverb

Most of the important things in the world have
been accomplished by people who have kept on
trying when there seemed to be no hope at all.
—Dale Carnegie

Pueblos of the American Southwest are the traditional
home communities of indigenous peoples. Some of these
locations have been continuously occupied for over a
thousand years, making them the oldest cities within
what is now the United States. They have survived fam-
ines, droughts, climate change, disease, and genocidal
violence, including the death and destruction perpe-
trated by conquistadors who were determined to displace
old languages and traditions and force new ones on the
pueblo dwellers. Ultimately, Catholicism was assimi-
lated, and adobe churches now stand above the ground,
complementing the underground kivas where native religion and traditions endure. On the pueblos today there
remains a communal sense of continuity and resilience.
"We are still here."

Most pueblo communities celebrate seasonal feast days, many of which are open to the public and usually include ceremonial dances enacted by tribal members, observances that can last for hours or days. Although southwestern precipitation tends to be sparse, averaging just 8–9 inches per year across large swaths of land, cloudbursts can occur, sending tourists scattering for shelter. The celebrants, however, continue dancing regardless of the weather.

Does hope inspire persistence, or does perseverance awaken hope? It's like the classic question of which came first, the chicken or the egg. Thoughts, feelings, and actions are intimately intertwined. In the preceding chapters we have considered facets of hope that are various blends of thinking and feeling, beliefs and emotions. Now we turn to *doing* as itself a form of hope. As author David Orr has observed, "Hope is a verb with its sleeves rolled up."

Action Prompts Hope

To persevere is to continue trying despite obstacles or opposition, to pursue what is difficult even after many optimists and realists have long since lost hope.[1] One might think that hope logically precedes and inspires action, and there is truth to this as we shall see later in the chapter. It is also true, however, that perseverance is itself an active form of hope. Endurance not only bespeaks but enacts hopefulness.

Perseverance is different from perseveration, which is merely continuing to do the same thing that isn't working. A popular saying in 12-step groups is that "Insanity is doing the same thing over and over again and expecting different results." Frustrated by patients' nonadherence to their advice, doctors sometimes complain that *I*

tell them and I tell them and I tell them and they still don't change!
Perhaps it's the *telling*, the *way* of advising that is the problem, and
a more collaborative approach could have better results.[2] When one
approach is not working, perseverance involves keeping an eye on
the horizon and trying out different paths to reach the destination
you desire. In his autobiography *Long Walk to Freedom,* Nelson
Mandela commented that "part of being optimistic is keeping one's
head pointed toward the sun, one's feet moving forward. There were
many dark moments when my faith in humanity was sorely tested,
but I would not and could not give myself up to despair. That way
lays defeat and death." Continuing to put one foot down in front of
the other is an act of hope.

Such tenacity is often rewarded. Instead of interpreting ineffective efforts as failures, you can understand them as *tries*. People
who try to stop smoking, for example, normally go through several
serious quit attempts before finally escaping nicotine addiction. In
making large or even small life changes it is unsurprising that any
single try does not suffice. Aspiring actors and cold-call salespeople
normally encounter many turndowns
before getting to a yes. The very act of
trying is a form of hope. Barack
Obama observed that "The best way
to not feel hopeless is to get up and do something. Don't wait for
good things to happen to you. If you go out and make some good
things happen, you will fill the world with hope, you will fill yourself with hope." That requires of course believing that you *can* succeed.[3] Actions are intended to effect something and thereby
embody hope. Continuing to try is a hopeful act.

In contrast, repeated experiences of futility can lead to learned
helplessness, a belief discussed in Chapter 5 that there is no point in

even trying.[4] This may be a generalized belief about powerlessness in life or it can be specific to particular situations. Learned helplessness has been demonstrated with laboratory animals and resembles the human experience of clinical depression.[5] In contrast, patient *activation* in health care encourages people to take a personal role in their own wellness and recovery.[6] An effective treatment for depression known as *behavioral activation* encourages people to engage in potentially pleasant activities even and especially when they do not feel like it, which in turn can evoke a positive mood.[7] In this way, emotions can be a result rather than merely a cause of what you do. Engaging in potentially pleasant activities precedes the lifting of depression and begins to restore hopefulness.

Proactive effort can also decrease adverse outcomes. A motivational interview with college students who had failed a first exam significantly increased their subsequent study behavior and eventually their grade, preventing course failure.[8] Behavioral activation interventions can reduce the occurrence of future depression or other major mental disorders.[9] Once again, taking action gives rise to hope.

There are complex cause-and-effect relationships among feeling, thinking, and doing, with each influencing the others. The point here is that actions can elicit both emotion and hope. In the language of ancient wisdom, "endurance produces character, and character produces hope."[10]

Hope Promotes Action

Hope, in turn, can motivate action. A classic metaphor is the carrot dangling from a string at the end of a stick, designed to motivate a donkey to move forward. In modern usage the stick in this image is often misrepresented as the threat of physical punishment (beating the animal), but the purpose of the stick is simply to suspend the carrot just beyond reach as a positive horizon toward which to move. If the donkey never actually received a carrot to eat, learned helplessness would likely set in.

At work or school, people with higher hope are more likely to do what is needed to succeed.[11] This is due in part to the fact that higher-hope employees or students behave in a characteristically different way when encountering obstacles. They look for new ways to reach their goal, whereas lower-hope people are more likely to give up.[12] In physical rehabilitation following an injury, a stroke. or surgery, patients with higher hope regain more functioning.[13] I have two friends who suffered devastating brain injuries and who, through dogged perseverance, managed to recover precious functions that most of us take for granted. I asked them how they had sustained hope to keep going on this arduous journey. A first response was "sheer stubbornness"—refusal to give up. There were also some little mental habits that helped, like including the concept of "yet" when thinking or talking about their recovery.

- I'm not able to use a cell phone *yet*.
- *So far* it's hard for me to talk to more than two or three people at a time.
- I'm *working up to* being able to ride my bicycle for two miles.

They reconceived obstacles as challenges. The modeling and support of others in recovery was also important. "If she can do it, so can I."

Hope may be expressed as a *promise*. The act of promising offers assurance and hope for the future to the extent that the person making it is judged to be trustworthy. Your own persistence can be strengthened by publicly stating your intention, as is formalized in an oath or a legal contract that requires it.[14] In traditional wedding vows, couples have made a far-reaching commitment to persist in loving each other "for better for worse, for richer for poorer, in sickness and in health, till death us do part." These now familiar words were penned by Thomas Cranmer, the Archbishop of Canterbury, in the 1549 English *Book of Common Prayer* as a liturgy for the new protestant Church of England. There is irony in the fact that this is the same archbishop who helped Henry VIII annul his first marriage and then presided over his subsequent weddings. However, Cranmer did not write the book until after Henry's death, so perhaps he conceived these wedding vows partly in response to his experience of the king's six marriages. Ultimately Cranmer himself was burned at the stake as a religious heretic.

Just as demoralizing experiences can result in learned helplessness, so also empowering experiences can foster learned hopefulness.[15] More active than broad optimism (Chapter 5), learned hopefulness applies problem-solving skills to gain perceived or actual control in aspects of your life, akin to the internal locus of control discussed in Chapter 3. You may take it for granted that you are able to make choices that influence your future, but it hasn't always been so. In ancient Greece, for example, people assumed that the gods predetermined their fate, and aspirational hope was therefore considered to be foolhardy *hubris*.[16]

Resilience

Adverse childhood experiences can predispose one to addiction, psychological disorders, educational underachievement, and conflicts with the law, but not necessarily. People can also survive a traumatic early life and thrive. Consider this woman's example. She was just 2 years old when her father violently murdered her mother. He evaded arrest, claiming that his wife had committed adultery and that his daughter was therefore illegitimate. The father quickly rewed, and when he died 12 years later her stepmother married a man who would sexually abuse the young girl, until finally she was sent away at 15 to live with relatives. By 20 she had been arrested and imprisoned, charged with a capital crime. Such an early history would not seem to bode well for her future, yet she was released from prison and at age 25 was crowned Elizabeth I, who became one of Europe's longest-reigning and most distinguished monarchs.

Then there's Joanne. When she was born, her working-class parents were just 19 years old. Her teachers pronounced her a "dunce" in primary school and "not exceptional" in secondary school. She married young and had a daughter with her abusive husband, who later divorced her. Joanne lost the office job that supported them and found herself a single mother struggling to get by on welfare benefits. She was depressed and suicidal. A year later she finished writing the first of the Harry Potter books that would ultimately sell more than 600 million copies, making J. K. Rowling one of the world's wealthiest women.[17]

Resilience or "grit" is the ability to adapt and thrive despite significant hardship.[18] Instead of being immobilized by stress, such people bounce back with confidence, optimism, and persistence.[19] A key seems to be how they respond to setbacks. A safe way to avoid inevitable disappointments is to lower your expectations and stop trying. In contrast, resilient people as individuals or leaders respond to hindrance by continuing to put forth effort even in the face of increasing adversity. When confronting problems they explore new

paths, confident in their ability to succeed eventually.[20] Martin
Luther King Jr. admired those who "have carved a tunnel of hope
through the dark mountain of disappointment."[21] You probably
know some remarkably resilient people, for they are many.

Perseverance: An Extended Story

Most of the stories in this book are short, but this one deserves
more space. It illustrates how hope promotes action, and action in
turn consolidates hope.

One of the most resilient people I have ever met is Debbie
Johnson, whose story exemplifies perseverance. We met at a gather-
ing for agencies and volunteers serving the homeless. She exuded
lovingkindness and energetic passion to serve women who had
experienced homelessness as she had. When I interviewed her for
this book 10 years later it was in the offices of the TenderLove
Community Center that she founded and directed. We silenced
our phones, but hers kept vibrating every few minutes, a testament
to the number of people eager to talk with her. The wall of her
office is full of awards and honors, not to mention a recently earned
master's degree in public health. Nothing there discloses her long
and difficult journey to the present.

Debbie was born to Christian parents in Ile-Oluji, Nigeria.
During college she became pregnant as an unmarried woman and
gave birth to a boy who was raised by her parents. She moved to
Nigeria's largest city, Lagos, intending to marry her son's father, but
things did not happen as they had planned. One day she returned
to the apartment they shared to find herself locked out, "ghosted"
in current parlance. As a single woman, she first supported herself

by working in a private elementary school, teaching science and cultural studies. She completed 2 further years of training as a nurse and began working in hospitals, where her passion to help people collided head-on with the economic realities of a health care system that required patients to pay before receiving even life-saving treatment. As she watched patients beg for care and die because of inability to pay, her compassion persuaded her that she had to find a different kind of work.

That's when she received an invitation from her American uncle to attend a family wedding and stay with him and his wife in Indiana. Never having been outside Nigeria, she obtained a visitor visa and arrived in Indianapolis in August of 2001, just a month before the 9/11 terrorist attacks on New York and Washington. Her visa was approved for 6 months, but in October her family told her that she could no longer stay with them, and she suddenly found herself homeless, facing a midwestern winter. "I had never seen snow before." A night job cleaning toilets in offices allowed her to sleep in a company van and apply for a Social Security number. She volunteered time at a Nigerian-founded church ministering to the homeless and managed to save enough money to get an apartment and a Dodge Neon, teaching herself to drive.

Debbie moved to the warmer climate of Atlanta, Georgia, working 12-hour shifts on two hospital jobs that often had her working 36 consecutive hours. She married, had two daughters, obtained a permanent resident card, continued working to support her family, and again volunteered at a church feeding homeless people. "What struck me there was that we kept seeing the same people over and over, people like me, and I began wondering how I could help them be able to support themselves." Debbie had also studied fashion design for 2 years while working in Nigeria, and she has a talent for sewing with or without patterns. "I began thinking that I could teach women how to sew and support themselves." She made a decision, reminiscent of Amelia Earhart's comment that "the most difficult thing is the decision to act, the rest is merely tenacity." She registered a nonprofit corporation for this purpose in Georgia but found little business support for herself as an African American woman, so she began searching online for locations where she could serve a diverse population, helping women escape from poverty. "I had never seen a city with such a long name (Albuquerque) that I couldn't spell or pronounce, but it felt right." So in October of 2011 she packed up her sewing machines and fabric along with her family in a U-Haul truck and headed for New Mexico.

While working in hospitals and acute care centers, Debbie spent 2 years just learning about the Albuquerque community and existing programs. "I never wanted to compete with or duplicate services." She saw women sleeping under bridges and holding signs pleading for help. A particularly underserved population was recently incarcerated women, who were often being released from jail and dropped off downtown in the middle of the night. She moved the registration of her nonprofit center to New Mexico, and in 2013 rented a small building to begin teaching women how to sew. That's when I met her. The women had so many needs, some coming directly from jail with nothing more than the clothes they were wearing. There were programs in the city where they could get meals, but many of the women had no place to live, no job skills, little education, no transportation or even identification documents. Most were the sole head of their household, often with dependent children. What impressed me was Debbie's personal attention to these women, mentoring them for a year or more, which is the sort of sustained support and guidance needed to escape the bonds of poverty. I have worked in large agencies serving thousands of people, but the smaller, intimate atmosphere of the TenderLove Community Center touched me. "I just decided not to give up," Debbie said. "From where we were, I could see the future. I don't believe something is impossible."

Within half a year the group had outgrown the space. A feature story on a local television channel attracted enough support to let them move to a larger building across town. My primary contribution was teaching Debbie how to organize and write grant proposals for funding, and she was a quick study. I also helped her start collecting consistent data about her clients and eventually to conduct a follow-up study of everyone who had graduated from the program over a 3-year period. An astonishing 97 percent of them were in stable housing, with 88 percent employed and 9 percent enrolled in higher education. With support attracted from many sources, the group again outgrew its facility, moving to a still larger building with a storefront to sell the women's handiwork. Within a few years Debbie established a business called Sew4Real, where graduates could continue working together. She added training in computer and financial literacy, helped a number of women start their own businesses, and added not one but two houses where unhoused women and their children could live while working in the program to get into their own apartment.

And all through the first 10 years of the TenderLove program, Debbie served without salary as CEO of the program while working to make ends meet. In the early years she often pawned her car title for short-term loans to pay the bills and keep the facility open. She would spend her last dollar to help someone in need. She has endured financial hardship, the COVID-19 pandemic, disappointments, and personal heartbreak, always focused on empowering the vulnerable women in her program to become independent and dependable.

"How do you explain all that resilience and energy?" I asked her. Certainly her deep faith sustains her. "I just think of myself as a child of God, not in a particular religion," she said. "I go blindly with God. I trust that God will solve my problems while I am helping others solve theirs," and it seems to be true. On her office wall is a small saying, "When you pray for rain, take your umbrella." Her mother was an iron lady, deeply strong, who taught Debbie to be reliable and unselfish. "Mama cooked a large meal every morning, welcoming anyone around who was hungry. By the end of the day the food was gone, and the next morning she did it all again." Debbie just trusts that her good work will bear good fruit, and she keeps going. As I write this, she is happily enrolled and taking classes in a doctoral program in counseling and psychological studies.

Futile Persistence

Although perseverance can be rewarded and statistically improbable hopes are also sometimes realized by happenstance or self-fulfilling prophecy, there are also times when persistence is fruitless. The original "serenity prayer" mentioned in Chapter 3 asks for "courage

> Can you think of a time in your life when you kept trying too long, too often, too hard to make something happen?

to change what must be changed, serenity to accept what cannot be helped, and the insight to know the one from the other." The discernment here is between truly false hopes and those that are achievable with perseverance.

Unsuccessful efforts often cause people to dial down their expectations, and continuing to try can yield disappointment, stress, frustration, and depletion of resources.[22] A spectacular example of inappropriate persistence is the first attempt to construct the Panama Canal.[23] The French diplomat Ferdinand de Lesseps, who had successfully negotiated construction of the Suez Canal, was subsequently assigned to encore his celebrated feat by connecting the Atlantic and Pacific oceans across the Isthmus of Panama. He was determined to dig the canal at sea level as had been done successfully before, but the rainforest jungle terrain proved quite different from the desert of Egypt. After a decade of laborious digging on a massive scale, disastrous landslides, and tropical diseases that killed many thousands of workers, the project was finally abandoned. The canal was ultimately completed 25 years later by finding a new approach to the goal: a series of locks to raise ships about 85 feet from one ocean and lower them down to the other. Here is an illustration of the difference between perseveration (persisting with the same unsuccessful strategy) and perseverance (continuing efforts that include trying new avenues to reach a destination).

Apparent futility sometimes evokes inspiring individual protests, like the anonymous man facing down a line of tanks in Tiananmen Square or Vedran Smailović and his cello sailing Albinoni's Adagio into the empty air amid the bombed-out streets of Sarajevo. Once, for unknown reasons, many whales beached themselves on the Oregon coast and lay dying in the sand. A Portland TV station that day aired a video of a small child traversing the beach, methodically carrying pails of water from the sea to pour on each whale. It was heartbreakingly hopeless. It was timeless.[24]

Even when unfulfilled, hopes may have some beneficial effects and unanticipated consequences. Hope can hold adversity at bay, encouraging endurance and creative adaptation. A 19th-century Vermont farmer named William Miller (no relation) became convinced, based on biblical study, that the world would come to an end on a particular date in 1843. He began preaching and amassed many followers who were called Millerites or Adventists. When the predicted cataclysm failed to materialize, various explanations emerged for the disappointment, including that the expected event had actually occurred on schedule, but had happened in heaven rather than on earth. The Millerite movement endured and continued to grow, eventually becoming the Seventh-day Adventist Church, which now claims 20 million adherents worldwide.

The idea that hope can be "false" arises from thinking of hope in a rather limited way, namely as the realistic probability that something will happen (Chapter 3). The facets of hope we have considered thus far range well beyond statistical likelihood to perceiving possibilities and purpose as well as mobilizing desire, optimism, and trust. Things are impossible until they're not, and perseverance is itself a facet of hope. Besides all this, there can also be a hope beyond hope.

TAKING IT PERSONALLY: PERSEVERANCE

- Does it seem like a strange idea that *doing* something is a facet of hope? Which seems truer to you: that hope leads to action or that action fosters hope?

- What do you think helps people become more resilient? What has helped you persevere?

- When might "Just do it!" be good advice to do something that you don't feel like doing?

CHAPTER 9

Hope beyond Hope

"Hope sees the invisible, feels the intangible,
and achieves the impossible."
—Helen Keller

"I've always had a weakness for lost causes,
once they're really lost."
—Rhett Butler in the film *Gone with the Wind*

In the summer before my senior year at Lycoming College, a group of students and faculty traveled to nearby Bucknell University to hear the Czech Philharmonic Orchestra during its U.S. tour. It was August of 1968, and as it happened, on the very day of their scheduled concert Soviet tanks were rolling into Czechoslovakia to crush liberalization reforms of the Prague Spring. We wondered whether the orchestra would still perform given the unexpected chaos at home, but play they did. A centerpiece of the program was Má Vlast (My Country), a cycle of six symphonic poems written a century earlier by the Czech composer Bedrich Smetana to celebrate his homeland and culture. The orchestra performed it with astonishing passion that evening, a fervor that I still recall whenever I hear it. They played into the air of the concert hall their hope and vision for their nation's future. The occupation would continue for 23 years before the troops finally withdrew and the independent Czech Republic was born with an artist as its president: the author and poet Vaclav Havel, who had earlier written from prison that "The most important thing of all is not to lose hope and faith in life itself. Anyone who does so is lost."[1]

There is yet another hope beyond all of the facets considered thus far—after probability and possibility, desire and optimism; beyond trust, meaning, and perseverance. It has been called hope against hope or, as I chose to title this chapter, a hope beyond hope, one that remains and sustains us when all of the more familiar ways of hoping seem to be exhausted.[2] Such ultimate hope endures beyond hardships, danger, and suffering, even to the end of life itself. It is not a belief or an emotion so much as a commitment to a vision. Ultimate hope seeks to keep faith with deeply held values and without regard or attachment to immediate outcomes. It is a conviction that something better is ultimately possible for us collectively.[3] In Vaclav Havel's words, it is hope and faith in life itself.

We are entitled to keep on hoping when finite hopes are dashed.[4] This ultimate, nonrational kind of hope can be a matter of life and death, particularly when the future seems bleak.[5] The alternative is hopelessness, a common companion of depression and suicide. Fyodor Dostoevsky warned that "to live without hope is to cease to live," and Charles Dickens urged, "Don't leave off hoping, or it's of no use doing anything. Hope, hope to the last." In the more poetic language of Gabriel Marcel, "Hope is for the soul what breathing is for the living organism. Where hope is missing, the soul dries up and withers."[6]

A harrowing account of hope against hope is that of the Dougal Robertson family, who were shipwrecked with four children far out at sea in the Pacific when their boat was damaged by a pod of whales and sank. Left with few supplies in a 10-foot wooden lifeboat, their group of six survived for 38 days on fish and rainwater before being sighted and rescued. "Even if you give up hope," Robertson wrote, "you must never give up trying, for, as the result of your efforts, hope may well return and with justification."[7]

Hope beyond hope does have some commonalities with other facets that we have considered. Like all hope, it envisions the possibility of a brighter future, if only for generations to come, and can inspire persistent action toward that hoped-for vision without any reasonable expectation of success. Hope beyond hope may include a trust in ultimate benevolence or a purposive commitment, come what may, to the selfless form of loving to which world religions point.[8] Some perceive a benign ultimate destination toward which history steadily evolves.

The core characteristic of hope beyond hope is a refusal, regardless of current reality, to give up and succumb to hopelessness, cynicism, or despair. After more than 2 years of hiding in an attic with her Jewish family during the Nazi occupation of Amsterdam, 16-year-old Anne Frank wrote in her now famous diary just 3 weeks before being arrested and sent to Auschwitz:

> In spite of everything I still believe that people are really good at heart. I simply can't build up my hopes on a foundation consisting of confusion, misery, and death. I see the world gradually being turned into a wilderness, I hear the ever approaching thunder, which will destroy us too, I can feel the sufferings of millions and yet, if I look up into the heavens, I think that it will all come right, that this cruelty too will end, and that peace and tranquility will return again.[9]

The imagery of such ultimate hope is often about light, without which nothing at all can be seen. Some familiar images are that:

It is always darkest just before the dawn.

Darkness is what allows us to see the stars.

It is better to light one candle than to curse the darkness.

Hope beyond hope is about perceiving light and, like a sunflower, turning toward it. It is something that arises in you to keep you going when other forms of hope seem to be gone.

Hope as Horizon

The light within hope beyond hope often appears as a horizon, a longed-for future toward which you face and move despite uncertainty and adversity. To his family during his 27-year imprisonment, Nelson Mandela wrote, "I am certain that one day I will be back at home to live in happiness with you until the end of my days," and so it would come to pass.[10] Yet this kind of ultimate hope does not need to assume that you will personally witness its realization. The horizon on which you fix your gaze may be far beyond your own lifetime. Holding to the horizon can be seen in planting trees that will never give you shade personally; recycling reusable materials; and writing letters, songs, or books that may have no apparent impact. You can take a long perspective, thinking ahead for generations or centuries. As mentioned in Chapter 1, the scientist–futurist Pierre Teilhard de Chardin confidently envisioned a meaning-filled universe that is ultimately converging toward a hopeful omega point.[11] Others envision that in the 21st century the world is already embarking on a *Great Turning* to

Hope beyond Hope 119

shift our ways of thinking, acting, and being toward life-sustaining change.[12]

The horizons toward which we face and move often evolve over the course of a lifetime. From a young age my own conviction was to become a pastoral minister, which was the primary motivation for being the first in my family to go to college. I majored in psychology, thinking that it would be useful for a pastor, and, at a deeper level, hoping to better understand my own muddled self. My career path subsequently shifted toward psychology as my calling with, as mentioned earlier, a particular passion to alleviate suffering related to alcohol and other drug use. I had not experienced addiction in my own family, but I had witnessed the long-term ravages of substance use in hospitalized patients and was persuaded to head upstream to find ways of helping people escape the currents of addiction before reaching the devastation awaiting them downstream. Understanding and treating addictions became a new horizon for me that eventually broadened into helping people get unstuck from destructive life patterns that ensnare them.[13] Finding myself in a professional doorway between psychology and spirituality, I began passing knowledge back and forth between these perspectives.[14] The ministry that I glimpsed early has continued to evolve.

Sometimes new horizons appear as dramatic insights or epiphanies.[15] English seaman John Newton worked on and later captained sailing ships that transported enslaved people from Africa. Then he himself was enslaved in Africa, and soon after being rescued found himself facing death aboard a ship foundering in a fierce storm at sea. Not a religious man, he nevertheless prayed to be delivered.[16] Arriving safely home, John refrained from drinking and gambling and eventually became an Anglican priest and ardent opponent of the slave trade. He lived to see the abolition of slavery in England and is most remembered for hymns that he wrote, including "Amazing Grace": "I once was lost but now am found, was blind but now I see." Both Leo Tolstoy and Fyodor Dostoevsky had sudden epiphanies that altered their understanding of life and shaped their future writing.[17] Such transforming events are often documented in autobiography as turning points that redirected the lives of people like Jane Addams, Malcolm X, Oscar Romero, and Siddhartha Gautama toward new meaning and purpose in life.

In a popular modern story, a boy is asked by a mole the question that is so often posed to children: "What do you want to be when you grow up?"[18] His answer is simple: "Kind." What is the light toward which you are drawn, the horizon toward which you hope to move? How can you live with integrity toward a value to which you aspire? Think of momentum with each choice that you make or action that you take. Does it move you toward your horizon or farther back from it? Using the analogy of a motor vehicle, are you in forward or reverse gear or perhaps more commonly in neutral and not moving at all? Every journey is spent in some combination of these gears. For example, here are 12 dimensions of lovingkindness with descriptions of forward, neutral, and reverse gears:[19]

FORWARD	NEUTRAL	REVERSE
Compassionate	Indifferent	Cruel
Empathic	Apathetic	Adversarial
Contented	Discontented	Envious
Generous	Self-centered	Greedy
Hopeful	Objective	Pessimistic
Affirming	Ignoring	Demeaning

Forgiving	Resentful	Vengeful
Patient	Impatient	Intolerant
Humble	Immodest	Arrogant
Grateful	Unappreciative	Entitled
Helpful	Unhelpful	Obstructive
Yielding	Unyielding	Dominating

On each dimension you can consider where you or others you know spend most of life. I consider these dimensions when pondering politicians who ask for my vote. It is possible to move along each dimension based on the daily choices that you make and actions you take. You could describe similar dimensions of forward, neutral, and reverse regarding other values to which you aspire.

What is the light toward which you are drawn, the horizon toward which you hope to move in your lifetime?

Horizons emerge not only for individuals, but also for groups of people as a movement.[20] In this way, hope can be collective and interpersonal rather than merely a solitary experience.[21] Groups and organizations can share common goals and perseverance in pursuing them even when there seems to be little chance of succeeding. The suffrage movement persisted in many nations for decades, eventually yielding the right to vote for women, first in New Zealand in 1893. A desire for national sovereignty has emerged in many independence movements, ranging from the 18th-century Boston Tea Party and the French Revolution, to the Polish Solidarity movement and African nations' independence movements in the 20th century, and Britain's "Brexit" from the European Union in 2020. Social movements diminished racial segregation in the United States and South Africa and changed civil and LGBTQ+ rights and abortion and capital punishment policies in many nations.

According to historian Howard Zinn, a common and ironic characteristic of successful social movements is that they often begin from hopelessness![22] At the outset they appear to be lost causes—abolishing slavery, instituting universal suffrage, and realizing civil rights—with little chance of seeing the hoped-for change in one's lifetime.

A classic example of hope beyond hope is the 2,800-year-old vision of abolishing war and other forms of violence that is inscribed on a sculpture gifted to the United Nations by the Soviet delegation in 1959:

> *They shall beat their swords into ploughshares, and their spears into pruning hooks; nation shall not lift up sword against nation, neither shall they learn war any more.* [23]

Such ultimate hope for nonviolence is central in the teachings of Jesus, Gandhi, and Dr. King, all of whom lived to the end the values for which they would ultimately be martyred, refusing to return hate for hate, violence for violence.

There can be value in dreaming a seemingly impossible dream despite the evidence. Rather than acceding to helplessness, such imagining affirms that the world is malleable and envisions how change would look or could occur.[24] Instead of waiting for a sudden worldwide cessation of violence, we can seek a deeper understanding of its causes and begin working now on a different way of being together. There are many forms of aggression short of physically harming someone, such as passive–aggressive behavior and psychological abuse. Indirect,

> What is an important value that you hope to represent in your own life? During the past year, how much time have you spent in forward, neutral, and reverse gears with regard to this value?

subtle, even unintentional actions that exclude certain individuals or groups have been called *microaggressions*. There are also private internal experiences that can predispose us to antagonism toward others. Consider subjective attitudes and experiences such as these:

- Holding on to a grudge or resentment
- Being jealous or envious
- Desiring victory or revenge
- Delighting in another's frustration or downfall
- Feeling superiority and self-satisfaction
- Being certain of your correctness
- Ridiculing, dismissing, or excluding others

These are all rooted in comparing oneself with others, which readily gives rise to vanity or resentment. We can notice these potential roots of antagonism when we experience them and do the inner work of peacemaking. It's a hope-beyond-hope step toward how things could and ought to be. Although ending violence may be a remote dream, nonviolence can begin with changing our own behavior and attitudes.[25]

To Wait with Hope

In Spanish the same verb, *esperar,* means both to wait and to hope. Both waiting and hoping face toward the future. Hopeful waiting is the essence of a vigil or a period of preparation. The waiting may be inspired by a particular expectation, such as the hope of permanent residency for immigrant "Dreamers" who were brought to the United States as undocumented children. This waiting *for* something is perhaps the most common association with both hoping and waiting. Even with a specific desired outcome, hope may involve simply waiting with trust and anticipation when nothing more can be done. Such is the hopeful waiting for news of a missing pet or person.

However, there is also a form of hope beyond hope that has no specific goal, like music without words—a hope beyond particular objects or outcomes. There is nothing wrong with waiting *for* something, but in an age of instant information and gratification, simply waiting without specific expectations is a nearly lost art.

When we were living in Sydney, Australia, for a year, I would walk each morning up a long, grassy hill from Coogee Beach to Randwick. My normal routine was to turn left at the top of the hill and stroll through town to the addiction research center where I was working. Along the way I had often noticed a large Catholic church perched atop the hill and off to the right. One morning as I climbed the hill I felt an odd inclination to go into the church, which I had never visited. It didn't make any sense, but the urging grew, and so when I reached the top I turned right. The door was open, the sanctuary quiet and empty, so I found a pew off to one side and sat down. I slowed my breathing and settled into a meditative state. Ten minutes, 20, and the word that I felt was *Wait!* So I sat in silence. *For what?* I wondered, but the word was still *Wait!* A few other people came in and out. I thought about what I had planned to do that day with nothing on my schedule. *How long should I remain here?* And again a clear *Wait!* No one knew where I was, and perhaps someone would begin to wonder. *Really? How long? All morning? Through lunch? All day? Wait for what? What if my wife tries to call me?* This was before cell phones. She would worry. I struggled with the irrationality of it. *Wait!* I knew that well more than an hour had passed. Morning light fell through the air, which still smelled of incense. More silence. *All right,* I thought at last, *I don't understand. This is crazy. It doesn't make any sense to me, but if you want me to wait here, then I will, as long as it takes.* And immediately came the reply as clearly as if it had been spoken: *OK, you can go now.* I laughed aloud.

There is an ancient contemplative discipline of opening the mind and heart, focusing attention on your breath or a word or an object and silencing the monkey mind of constant inner chatter. Thoughts and feelings arise, but you don't follow them. You simply watch them pass by, like leaves floating along a quiet stream. It has been called *mindfulness meditation,* the *relaxation response,* and *centering prayer.*[26] There are widely studied health benefits, but it is a discipline of waiting with no expected outcome. In a witty cartoon by Gahan Wilson, two robed monks sit side by side in meditative posture, and the old one is saying to the younger, "Nothing happens next. This is it." Paying patient close attention without specific expectation is a countercultural practice in an achievement-oriented, results-focused information society where waiting is thought to be fruitless unless it leads to the desired outcome. Closely related to mindfulness is a form of deep empathic listening with no aim other than to understand another person's experience.[27]

There is even reason to wait before hoping. To wait with specific expectations can narrow your vision. In his poem "East Coker" within *The Four Quartets,* T. S. Eliot wrote:

> I said to my soul, be still, and wait without hope
> For hope would be hope for the wrong thing . . .
> The faith and the love and the hope are all in the waiting.

Hope beyond hope can be curious anticipation of and openness to experience, letting the unexpected happen.[28] Good science is like that: open-minded observation of whatever is. I remember a graduate student who came to my office just after analyzing the data from her master's thesis. "I didn't find anything," she despaired.

"Yes, you did," I replied. "You just didn't find what you expected."

Hope then can transcend even goals. It can endure beyond hoping *for*, as an existential state of mind and heart that anticipates an uncertain future with curiosity rather than fear. This is the hope beyond all other varieties of hope, captured so well by Emily Dickinson: *Hope is the thing with feathers that perches in the soul and sings the tune without the words and never stops at all.*

TAKING IT PERSONALLY: HOPE BEYOND HOPE

- When was the last time you simply waited quietly without waiting *for* anything?

- What is an example of hoping for something beyond your own lifetime that you yourself never expect to see?

- How might you describe a "faith in life itself"?

CHAPTER 10

Choosing Hope

Hope is the openness of love to infinite possibilities
and new life.

—ILIA DELIO[1]

"Where there's hope, there's life. It fills us with fresh
courage and makes us strong again."

—ANNE FRANK[2]

It was the hardest thing we had ever done. Our application process to become adoptive parents had required more than a year of clearing physical exams, psychological evaluations, background checks, home visits, and several interviews. Then it took several phone calls and more waiting before a state social worker finally came to our home with the big book of children available for adoption, a large binder in which each double-paged story spoke heartbreak. There were so many children in need of a good home, their photos looking out at us with half-hopeful smiles. Almost all of them were boys. We learned later that girls are far more likely to be taken in by relatives rather than turned loose for foster care or adoption. I felt the lonely reality that boys are more likely to be abandoned.

As I mentioned in Chapter 5, we eventually chose a brother and sister, ages 8 and 9, who had already experienced more abuse and trauma than anyone should have to endure in a lifetime. Unbeknown to us, their social worker had also chosen us from the book of potential parents, and within a few weeks they were living with us. The state required at least a year's waiting period of getting to know each other before an adoption could be finalized. We were novices as parents, of course, never having established house rules, meal routines, study habits, or bedtimes, all of which had to be developed, like building an airplane while flying it. They were children who had grown up without much structure or supervision, so all of this was new to them as well. They complained bitterly to our family therapist, "Who are these people trying to set rules and limits for us?" And to us they said, "We're nothing like you!" I once commented to our daughter that something she had said to a classmate sounded mean. "You don't know what mean is," she retorted, and the truth of it chilled me.

After a year we were both exhausted, worn down by everyday stress, conflict, and uncertainty. We felt hopeless, afraid that it would always be this way or worse. One Saturday, in despair, we privately concluded that parenting these children was too much for us, and we had to go back to the state to find a new home for them. The weight of failure and remorse was intense, and I wept that night as hard as I ever have, grieving both for them and for us. It was one of the worst moments of my life.

Sunday morning came, and as usual we went to the congregation that was our supportive extended family. As it happened, that morning there was a guest preacher, Pastor Jorge, from a sister church in Mexico, who spoke in Spanish with a translator standing beside him. His sermon text was the biblical story of a third appearance of Jesus after his death.[3] His broken-hearted disciples had left Jerusalem and gone back to their old familiar life as fishermen. All night they had fished in vain, catching nothing at all, and that's when they noticed a stranger on the shore who turned out to be their beloved teacher. "This time," Pastor Jorge said, "he is not in the holy city, but out in the everyday world of life and work. This story tells us that God is not merely found in holy spaces, but is with us in the hard places and in the midst of failure."

When the service was over, we walked out of the sanctuary together. "Did you feel like that was for us?" Both of us clearly did. We decided to keep on trying, to trust that in dark places we are not alone. It was enough. Adolescence was very long for us all, but our children are now grown with work and families of their own, and we have the added joy of knowing grandchildren and great-grandchildren.[4]

Hope and transformation can and do emerge from deep darkness, from the caverns of fear, anger, and despair.[5] What seems impossible becomes possible, and the irreconcilable can find resolution. One possibility is peaceful acceptance of present reality that this is just how it is going to be. In Niebuhr's words it's finding "the serenity to accept what cannot be helped."

Hope is quite a different resolution. It lifts our vision beyond the moment at hand toward a yet undetermined and potentially better horizon. It is a choice to remain open for new horizons rather than retiring to neverland. "Never" thinking closes down the future with dark hopelessness:

I'm never going to . . .

That's impossible.

I won't ever be able to . . .

It's never going to happen.

Hope is like the dawning of light, like drawing a fresh breath. It connects us to the malleable future that is forever becoming the present. When distress arises in the normal course of life, you can always choose to focus on hope in any of its varieties.

Acting on hope is vitally different from accepting the status quo or dwelling on distress. Even in the midst of the most dire of circumstances we can willingly choose hope. Viktor Frankl, a survivor of four Nazi death camps, wrote this:

> We who lived in concentration camps can remember the men who walked through the huts comforting others, giving away their last piece of bread. They may have been few in number, but they offer sufficient proof that everything can be taken from a man but one thing: the last of the human freedoms—to choose one's attitude in any given set of circumstances, to choose one's own way. . . . In the final analysis it becomes clear that the sort of person the prisoner became was the result of an inner decision, and not the result of camp influences alone.[6]

We live in a distressing, dismaying, even frightening world. Hope is a good way to live in that world. As discussed throughout this book, we have available to us a rich variety of ways for hoping. We can select among them, exploring the facets that best represent hope in present circumstances. We may not know in advance which aspects of hope are most fitting, but we can try them out, like flipping through an optician's lenses to discover what best brings the future into focus.

Let's reexamine the diamond of hope, revisiting its eight facets as choices we can make, not only when facing adversity, but also in daily life. With each facet, I suggest some questions to consider with regard to choosing hope.

Desire

In a story that has had many forms, we all hold inside us two animals that are always battling with each other. One of them is selfish, trying to take whatever it wants without regard for others. The second is also strong and willing to share territory and resources. They correspond roughly to the characters Scar and Simba in The Lion King, but this struggle is within us. The story always ends with an anxious question: "Which one is going to win?"—and an answer: "The one that you feed."

There is no hope without desire. What you choose to want, to wish for, matters. Wanting is a prerequisite for all kinds of hoping. In the language of the Pygmalion effect, what you deeply want affects what you both see and get. Of course you don't always get what you want, but desire changes the terrain, shaping the possibilities that you will perceive and influencing what will actually happen.

Desire is a matter of judged importance. We are surrounded by information (opinion, advertising, persuasion, preaching, and teaching) that is at least partially intended to influence what we regard to be important. To be sure, there are innate survival needs for air, water, and food as well as basic psychological needs for love, security, and belonging. Beyond these needs, your perceptions of what is important and how much you need of it are influenced by your social environment. Priorities about what matters are sometimes turned upside down by sudden epiphanies or a near-death experience.[7] Intentional reflection on your own values can help clarify what is most important.[8]

What you want and expect for others also matters. Hope only for oneself is a poor and self-centered desire. Hopes for those we know and love can become self-fulfilling prophecies. You can lend your hope to people who have none, who are indifferent or discouraged, even to those who would crush hope in others.[9] Keeping hope to yourself is of limited benefit.

It is also true that you don't have to pursue whatever you want. The restaurant server's question "Would you like some dessert?" anticipates but does not determine what you will actually choose. Sometimes a waiter presents an array of tempting dessert options to the table, urging you one step closer to a choice and away from saying "no thank you." A principle of temptation is that the physical proximity of desirable options can increase your wanting. Nevertheless, in answer to "Do you want dessert?" it is possible to answer, "Yes I do, and no thank you." You don't *have* to get what you want.

The ability to choose what you want may seem paradoxical. Isn't wanting just hardwired or conditioned, sometimes even unconscious? Yes, that is partially true, and trying *not* to want something is rather like trying not to think about raccoons. The harder you try, the more you fail. Being told that you can't have something tends to make it all the more enticing. As a person with diabetes, I am sometimes asked what I can or can't eat. The truth is that I *can* eat anything; I am *able* to, and health is in the balance of choice and consequences.[10] I found that if I told clients or children that they couldn't do something, they would quickly prove me wrong.

To a substantial extent you choose what you desire. Be intentional about what you decide to want for yourself and others.

- What matters to you? What is truly valuable?
- If you decided that you want to change what is important to you, how might you go about it?
- What's an example of a time when your wanting something important helped it to happen?

Probability

"What are my chances, Doctor?" It's a common if sometimes unspoken question when diagnosed with a life-threatening illness. Perhaps a number can be offered based on science and past experience, but often what we long to hear is that the chances are not zero. We may embrace even small prospects rather than neverland.

When considering treatment for a significant health problem, people do wonder about their chances for a successful outcome. In the 1980s our research group telephoned a number of alcoholism treatment programs to ask about their success rate. Some honestly said that they did not know, but many did quote a figure, the lowest of which was 80 percent, in which case we asked how they knew. No one had anything even approaching objective data. They too actually didn't know but were being hopeful with statistics.[11]

Definitions of success matter. With regard to alcohol and other drug problems, great advances have been made in defining and measuring treatment outcomes. What constitutes a success when someone is treated for their smoking or drinking? One criterion is continuous perfection: that the person never drinks or smokes again. Expecting perfection is a common reason for the failure of New Year's resolutions. It's called the rule violation effect:

the idea that once you have broken the rule you have nothing left to lose.[12]

Expecting perfection in treating chronic illnesses would yield grim success rates. How often will a person who is being treated for diabetes, hypertension, depression, or asthma never again experience symptoms or need treatment? A reasonable hope in treating such conditions is that symptomatic episodes will become fewer, farther between, and less severe. Those who treat such chronic illnesses are rarely asked for a success rate. In addiction treatment, however, there has been an unfortunate tendency to classify treated cases as either successes or failures. A statistical "survival curve" is sometimes used to measure outcomes: what percentage of people are still totally abstinent (versus "relapsed") after various lengths of time?[13] Among those treated for alcohol problems in the United States, about one-quarter abstain from alcohol for a year, which doesn't sound very hopeful. As mentioned in Chapter 3, what is often overlooked is that the remaining majority drink 87 percent less on average, which is clearly enough to make a substantial difference in their health and quality of life.[14] Contrary to public and sometimes professional gloom, most people do get better. Thinking of hope in all-or-none terms is misleading and unnecessarily discouraging.

We differ in how much attention should be given to facts and figures. Some people anxiously look for daily facts in the realm of politics or finance, while others avoid such information and think little about it. Some people avoid medical tests and checkups lest they receive bad news. When given a new diagnosis of a serious medical condition, would you want to know all about it or prefer not to know? Probability is only one facet of hope, but it's an important one to consider.

- How much do you pay attention to information about climate change? Why is that?
- What hopes or decisions lie ahead for you for which having more information might be helpful? What kind(s) of information would you choose to know?
- Are there potential sources of relevant information that you tend to avoid? Why?
- In hoping, how much do you trust or rely on factual information, intuition, feelings, values, and other people's opinions?

Possibility

"But isn't it possible, Professor, that . . . ?" It's a question that I soon came to expect when cross-examined in court by an attorney hoping to raise reasonable doubt about my testimony. Psychology is not an exact science, and I usually had to acknowledge that "Yes, I suppose it's possible, though unlikely." After all, even when the chances of something are slim, it's often still imaginable as a possibility. Lawyers who hire an expert witness, though, would usually prefer to have one whose testimony conveys certainty rather than probability. I had a relatively short career as a forensic psychologist.

Possibility is appealing, though people may place too much hope in small likelihood. It keeps casinos and lotteries in business, and sometimes it's quite understandable to choose possibility over probability.[15] What if the actual prospect of a successful life-saving surgery is only 5 percent? Chances are that you might still want to have the surgery for yourself or a loved one who otherwise would die.

Perceiving possibilities is a gift that you can offer to people, to an organization, or to a cause. The ability to envision different possibilities is fundamental to creativity and in mentoring. It was a gift that teachers gave to me, seeing potential that I had not envisioned myself. Sometimes a small encouragement of possibility can have major life impact. Before I had ever written an article or imagined doing so, Professor Lewis Goldberg encouraged me because he thought that a term paper I had written for his class was good enough to be in a scientific journal and should be. He coached me to submit it, and it became my first professional publication.[16] At a point in my life when I wasn't even clear what kind of work I hoped to do, that article helped me land a faculty post and begin a lifelong career as a psychology professor and writer. I in turn intentionally sought to envision and suggest possibilities for the students I mentored.

Not everyone wants to be seen as having potential. As mentioned in Chapter 4, the knight-errant Don Quixote in *The Man of La Mancha* meets a prostitute named Aldonza whom he envisions and treats as the noble Lady Dulcinea. She angrily rails at him that of all the men who had abused her, he was actually the cruelest of all by offering her false hope.[17] Nevertheless, by the story's end, she embodies and restores Don Quixote's own lost vision.

You can choose to look for, envision, and impart possibilities. I had a friend who truly disliked his job, but was so uncommonly good at perceiving possibilities that his company kept on raising his salary to keep him. He was too valuable to lose, though ultimately his own envisioned possibility of a more rewarding line of work won. He quit his job, retrained, and decades later continues to enjoy his work although he could retire. Possibility-hope reaches beyond present reality and probabilities.

- What possibilities do you see for you to make a modest contribution in solving a major social problem today?
- How might a workplace or organization of which you are a part encourage people to envision and communicate different possibilities?
- What established routines are there in your life, work, or family that could use some refreshing new options?

Optimism

Optimism and pessimism are chosen perspectives. Either one can be rationalized but not proven to others, and both may be regarded by the holder as realism. They are essentially default assumptions: When there is doubt or ambiguity, is it more likely that the eventual outcome will be good or bad? The phrase "benefit of the doubt" describes an optimistic default stance. If a friend or lover isn't answering the telephone, immediately entertained explanations may be optimistic: that they are busy, sleeping, relaxing, or shopping, or perhaps their cell phone battery is depleted or they have forgotten to turn the phone on. Pessimistic guesses (suspicious doubt) could be jumping to the conclusion that the person is angry, intentionally refusing to answer, is avoiding or snubbing you, or even is ill or has died. No assumption immediately alters or clarifies why the person isn't answering. Benefit versus suspicion of the doubt, though, may influence how you feel and think in the meantime and also what you say when next you meet.

The consequences of optimism or pessimism for you, the guesser, are more consistent. The choice of assumptions affects not only how you feel in the moment, but also influences longer-term health and relationships. Such chosen explanations can make themselves come true. As discussed in Chapter 5, pessimism is associated with a plethora of medical, psychological, and interpersonal ills. Choose benefit of the doubt! You can double down with active optimism, doing something to fulfill the positive expectation rather than sitting back passively and waiting.

You may have doubts about choosing optimism, particularly if you lean toward pessimism and you hate being disappointed. I sometimes describe myself as a pathological optimist. I choose to err on the side of trusting, forgiving, trying too long, and expecting the best in people. Disappointment doesn't often sting me much, and "until proven otherwise" may take a bit too long for me. Still I think it's worth the risk. Unwarranted pessimism can be more costly than unearned optimism.

There is a well-developed science of replacing hopeless and self-defeating thoughts.[18] In simplistic terms, a first step is to catch yourself thinking negatively and to recognize that you are making assumptions. What is it that you are telling yourself in situations of doubt and uncertainty? A next step is to interrupt the habit; for example, by telling yourself something like "now wait a minute...." Then find a replacement or antidote thought to fill the uncertainty with a more optimistic possibility. It's a matter of practicing a new way of thinking that gives yourself and others the benefit of the doubt.

- How conscious are you that in situations of doubt or uncertainty, your thoughts are actually guesses?
- Can you think of a situation in which you assumed the worst, and you turned out to be wrong?

- What line of reasoning could you offer to yourself or someone else for giving the benefit of the doubt?
- If you were to decide to adopt a more optimistic attitude, what might be a first step?

Trust

I remember one night leaving a remote building in an unfamiliar part of town where I had just given a lecture. It was a moonless night, and the parking lot was unlighted as I walked toward my car at some distance from the building. As my eyes began adjusting to the darkness, I heard footsteps coming up behind me. My pace quickened, and so did the footsteps as well as my heart rate.

"Dr. Miller?" Oh, a relief; it's someone who knows me. I stopped and turned to learn who it was, with an upward blip in trust. He was a big fellow, like a football player.

"You may not remember me," he said, "but I was a student at the university a few years ago and took your class on alcoholism." A bit more familiarity and trust.

"Oh, how was that class for you?"

"You gave me an F, and I flunked out of school." I felt renewed apprehension, heart rate back up again. I could barely make out his features in the dark, but I didn't remember him from a large lecture hall. People who took my alcoholism class often came with personal experience and pain. He may have been one of those who lined the back wall.

"Well, I hope that there was at least something useful in it for you."

"Oh, there was. I just wanted to thank you. Your course saved my life, and I'm 3 years sober now." Once again, relief.

"Congratulations! 3 years!" We shook hands, and then he gave me a bear hug.

Of all the kinds of hope considered in this book, trust may be the clearest example of a choice. No one decides for you whether you will trust, and it is an assessment that can fluctuate even from moment to moment. This brief example illustrates how trust and its opposite, fear, can oscillate within seconds.

Trust is a judgment about safety, assuming or entrusting your well-being with a person or situation. There are surely contexts in which trust is unwise. Increasingly clever scams arrive via the telephone and internet, warranting caution. Hypervigilance has survival value for soldiers in combat zones. On transition back to civilian life, whether from combat or prison, continuing hypervigilance is often part of post-traumatic stress, and it is a challenge to learn to trust again or perhaps for the first time.

Trusting involves courage and risk, but there are good reasons to choose and practice this form of hope. Just as mistrust is contagious, so trusting invites and provides an opportunity for trustworthiness. As we easily tend to be charitable regarding our own virtues and foibles, we can extend similar generosity to others. It is reasonable to trust and verify and also to accept and forgive. Do you know the aphorism that when you point a finger at someone else there are three fingers pointing back at you? Fault finding and judgment are easy; trusting is harder. It is my experience that when we practice acceptance of people just as they are, two interesting things occur. First, it makes it easier for them to change, and second, we become more accepting of our own shortcomings.

- What do you think and feel about choosing trust as a default starting assumption in relationships?
- What cues do you think influence you in deciding whether to trust or mistrust someone on first meeting?
- How might you experiment with offering trust and benefit of the doubt?

Meaning and Purpose

Whatever may be happening, you choose how you will understand it. You construct and discover meaning in life events be they joyful or distressing. Some people, for example, perceive the present as unfolding in accordance with an underlying benevolent plan or have a sense of personal purpose and mission in life that transcends specific events.[19] A sense of gratitude can provide a larger framework for experiencing life and death.[20] A frequent theme in mystical and transformational experiences is interconnectedness with all of humankind or a unity with all that is. Practicing mindfulness teaches acceptance without judgment. These perspectives are like a lens through which you experience and understand life. We can don such lenses but cannot prove or choose them for others. They are filters like those used to protect your eyes while viewing an eclipse of the sun.

For some people, a new lens on life happens in a momentary "aha" experience. They come to see life in a different way from their usual assumptions. Here's how one man described such an experience:

The whole thing came together for me, where I realized that there is a universal whole and through it I'm tied to

you and to everything in the universe. I saw that there's
something much greater than this physical world that we
live in, and I started asking, "What is real, what is the
meaning of life, what should I strive for?" I realized that
what was in my mind had been distorted, that as a kid I
was formed into something that my natural self wasn't. It
hit me that I was tied together with all those people I had
crunched and bulldozed along the way, and that being
kind to them was superimportant.[21]

I am grateful to be part of a men's support group that has been
meeting for more than 40 years. We gather every 2 weeks or so to
talk about what is happening in our lives. This group is for me
an invaluable lens to perceive meaning. These are guys who have
known me for such a long time that they understand the larger context within which current events enter into my life. Together we
have been through joy and grief, births and deaths, adoption and
separation, marriage and divorce. Countless times they have helped
me keep life experiences in larger perspective. This is a gift that
long-time friends can offer each other, listening well to how the
present is enfolded within the past and future.

Across cultures, having positive social relationships is linked
to happiness, well-being, and a sense of meaning in life.[22] Beyond
relationships, people also find meaning and purpose through work,
faith, and personal values. Life review and reminiscence are used
in many cultures to strengthen a sense of meaning, coherence, and
well-being and to alleviate depression and confusion in later years.[23]
Re-viewing and contemplating life events, for example in a gratitude diary, can also enhance meaning in life among young adults as
well.[24] Common in all of this is taking time to reflect on your life
experiences alone or in the company of others.

- What aspects of your own sense of meaning and purpose in life most give you hope?
- Sometimes meaning and purpose come with devotion to a particular person, value, or cause. To what or whom are you devoted?
- With whom have you shared enough years of life to reflect back on what it has meant to you individually and together?

Perseverance

Christine awoke in an intensive care bed 2 days after the head-on crash that severed her spinal cord leaving her paraplegic. There were days of foggy consciousness and confusion along with surgery to stabilize her back before she was moved to a recovery ward. Those visiting her on Saturday were surprised to find her sitting upright in bed bolstered by pillows, apparently in good spirits and working away with her laptop and cell phone. Friends wondered in whispers whether she was suffering from denial about her condition. What she was doing, as it turned out, was redesigning the entryway to their home for accessibility and deciding how a spare bedroom could be converted into a work-at-home office space. She asked for specific measurements to lay out plans. Her wife, however, was not at all surprised. "That's just what she does. Confronted with difficulties she goes right to problem solving. She'll be fine."

The choice of whether to keep going or give up is a matter of hope. I remember fondly watching a small child, maybe 2 or 3 years old, trying to stay upright on an ice-skating rink. Boy or girl, I couldn't tell, for the child was hooded, gloved, and padded like a teddy bear.

With no adult hovering nearby, the child would take a few short strides, sit down, get back up, advance, fall, and rise up undeterred over and over again. There was no apparent frustration or self-consciousness, just steady progress.

It's not quite as simple as "hopeful people just keep going." It's true that some people are by nature more stubborn and persistent, disinclined to change course just because of difficulty, whereas others when meeting obstacles prefer to look for an easier path. Either disposition can be wise or hazardous depending on the situation. The wisdom to know the difference between what is and isn't feasible is no simple matter, and trying out possibilities can be an important part of discernment. Continuing to try is a characteristic of resilience. The doing, the trying is itself a form of hope, and dogged perseverance sometimes accomplishes what was believed to be impossible.

Another choice is to accept that the desired change is not going to happen and move on. People who are in a difficult relationship weigh this decision of whether to keep on trying. With one of my colleagues it seemed that whatever I did in trying to smooth our relationship just made matters worse, and I finally decided that it was best to minimize contact. When the difficulties are with someone you love, it is challenging to set clear limits on what you will do and endure, while also preserving the cherished relationship. When efforts to reach a desired outcome are unsuccessful, lowering expectations is a normal response that also contains the risk of missing real opportunities.

Remember too the difference between perseveration and perseverance. In my career in the addiction field I met many people who had made multiple unsuccessful treatment attempts, sometimes 10 or more. It would be easy to conclude that such people are hopeless and will never change. Often what they had been offered was merely multiple rounds of the same treatment that hadn't worked for them. A general principle in health care is that when one approach isn't working, try something else. In treating behavioral health problems there is often a hopeful menu of different evidence-based alternatives. A compassionate system of care will make these various options available rather than requiring people to all fit into one kind of treatment.[25]

Choosing hope then can mean trying different approaches when something is not working. As described in Chapter 8, the deadly initial failure in building the Panama Canal was perseveration with one idea.

- When in your life have you kept on doing something that wasn't working?
- Think of someone from fiction or real life who kept trying different approaches to achieve a desired goal.
- What do you suppose keeps people hoping and going in spite of difficulties and obstacles? What keeps you going?
- How do you decide whether to persevere or accept what is?

Hope beyond Hope

No one can choose hope for you. People may tell you their own reasons for hoping, suggesting various viewpoints and alternatives, but ultimately the choice is yours. Similarly you can offer other people your own hopeful perspective, but the decision to receive it is theirs. You can show where the water is, but after that it's up to the drinker. Hope cannot be pushed in; it must be admitted and absorbed. That door opens from the inside.

We can choose to continue being hope-full even when other forms of hope seem to be exhausted. We can love without reservation or expectation.[26] We do not love our children only if they change, but *so that* they may change and grow. We choose the dawning horizon toward which to face our lives in hope.

Don't be discouraged by fluctuating or conflicting hope. That's normal. A hopeful state of mind is not perpetual but has peaks and valleys and at times falls silent altogether.[27] It is human to have conflicting hopes and feelings, and embracing them together can itself be a hopeful act. It is even possible to hold hope and despair simultaneously without having to choose between them.[28] As discussed in Chapter 9, we can choose to wait without expectation but still with a sense of expectancy, curiosity, and courage.

- What would you say are your deepest reasons for choosing hope?
- Do you know someone who retained hope against daunting odds, refusing to succumb to hopelessness, cynicism, or despair?
- What do you hold as an ultimate hope beyond your own lifetime?

Nurturing Hope

Finally, choose conditions that cultivate hope in yourself and others. There are at least these eight varieties of hope from which to choose. Use them like a palette of deep colors to paint your world.

Which of the aspects of hope considered in this book most easily find a home in you?

How are you choosing to hope (or not) right now in your life? You can decide what you want, what is most important (Chapter 2), imagining and exploring possibilities (Chapter 3). You can seek and be open to facts (Chapter 4) and accentuate the positive (Chapter 5). You can choose to give the benefit of the doubt (Chapter 6) and find hopeful meaning in what is (Chapter 7). Faced with disappointment and obstacles, you can opt to carry on or find new roads toward your destination (Chapter 8), and even when there seems to be no way forward you can will to keep faith with your values and vision (Chapter 9).

Conditions that foster hope in others also apply to you, and nourishing hope in others can energize your own.[29] When you are isolated, hopes are more difficult to find and maintain. Relationships and social support matter; hopeful birds flock together.[30] Become curious and explore together where hope may lie resting and how it can be awakened.[31] More than inaction, enacting hope even symbolically fuels empowerment.[32] Don't do nothing because you can only do a little. Even small tries can matter and are in themselves acts of hope.

Hope is how you address the present and the future that is forever becoming the present. When you have the opportunity, which is often, choose hope. Welcome it willingly. Seek hope in any of its many facets and you are likely to find it. In the end, choosing hope can be the most hopeful act of all.

So I leave you with a blessing from Nelson Mandela:

"May your choices reflect your hopes, not your fears."

Notes

CHAPTER 1. Finding Our Way in the Dark

1. Moltmann, J. (1993). *Theology of hope*. Fortress Press.
   Brueggemann, W. (2001). *The prophetic imagination* (2nd ed.). Fortress Press.
2. van Vliet, J. (2020). An ontology of human flourishing: Economic development and epistemologies of faith, hope, and love. In S. C. van den Heuvel (Ed.), *Historical and multidisciplinary perspectives on hope* (pp. 239–261). Springer Open.
3. From Alexander Pope (1734), *An essay on man*.
4. Wilkinson, R., & Pickett, K. (2009). *The spirit level: Why greater equality makes societies stronger*. Bloomsbury Press.
5. Webb, D. (2007). Modes of hoping. *History of the Human Sciences, 20*(3), 65–83.
6. 1 Corinthians 13:13. (1989). *The Holy Bible: New Revised Standard Version*. Oxford University Press.
7. Scioli, A. (2020). The psychology of hope: A diagnostic and prescriptive account. In S. C. van den Heuvel (Ed.), *Historical and multidisciplinary perspectives on hope* (pp. 137–163). Springer Open.
8. Kurin, R. (2007). *Hope diamond: The legendary history of a cursed gem*. HarperCollins.
9. Moltmann, J. (1993). *Theology of hope*. Fortress Press.
10. Boukala, S., & Dimitrakopoulou, D. (2017). The politics of fear vs. the politics of hope: Analysing the 2015 Greek election and referendum campaigns. *Critical Discourse, 14*(1), 39–55.

11. Tierney, J., & Baumeister, R. F. (2021). *The power of bad: How the negativity effect rules us and how we can rule it*. Penguin Books.

12. From a 1933 speech by President Franklin D. Roosevelt in the midst of the Great Depression.

13. Snyder, C. J. (2000). The past and possible futures of hope. *Journal of Social and Clinical Psychology, 19*(1), 11–28.

14. Beck, A. T., Steer, R. A., Beck, J. S., & Newman, C. F. (1993). Hopelessness, depression, suicidal ideation, and clinical diagnosis of depression. *Suicide and Life-Threatening Behavior, 23*(2), 139–145.

15. Haaga, D. A. F., & Beck, A. T. (1995). Perspectives on depressive realism: Implications for cognitive theory of depression. *Behaviour Research and Therapy, 33*(1), 41–48.

16. Shakespeare, W. *Hamlet*, Act III, Scene 1.

17. Menninger, K. (1959). The academic lecture on hope. *American Journal of Psychiatry, 116*(6), 481–491. Quotations from p. 481.

18. Schrank, B., Stanghellini, G., & Slade, M. (2008). Hope in psychiatry: A review of the literature. *Acta Psychiatrica Scandinavica, 118*(6), 421–433.

19. Goodall, J., Abrams, D., & Hudson, G. (2021). *The book of hope: A survival guide for trying times*. Celadon Books.
    Macy, J., & Johnstone, C. (2022). *Active hope: How to face the mess we're in with unexpected resilience & creative power* (rev. ed.). New World Library.
    Northcott, M. S. (2020). Ecological hope. In S. C. van den Heuvel (Ed.), *Historical and multidisciplinary perspectives on hope* (pp. 215–238). Springer Open.

20. van Vliet, J. (2020). An ontology of human flourishing: Economic development and epistemologies of faith, hope, and love. In S. C. van den Heuvel (Ed.), *Historical and multidisciplinary perspectives on hope* (pp. 239–261). Springer Open.

21. Olsman, E. (2020). Hope in health care: A synthesis of review studies. In S. C. van den Heuvel (Ed.), *Historical and multidisciplinary perspectives on hope* (pp. 197–214). Springer Open.
    Snyder, C. R., Irving, L. M., & Anderson, J. R. (1991). Hope and health. In C. R. Snyder & D. R. Forsyth (Eds.). *Handbook of social and clinical psychology: The health perspective* (pp. 285–305). Pergamon Press.

22. Duggleby, W., Hicks, D., Nekolaichuk, C., Holtslander, L., Williams, A., Chambers, T., & Eby, J. (2012). Hope, older adults, and chronic illness: A metasynthesis of qualitative research. *Journal of Advanced Nursing, 68*(6), 1211–1223.

Kylmä, J., Duggleby, W., Cooper, D., & Molander, G. (2009). Hope in palliative care: An integrative review. *Palliative and Supportive Care, 7*(3), 365–377.

23. Gravlee, G. S. (2020). Hope in ancient Greek philosophy. In S. C. van den Heuvel (Ed.), *Historical and multidisciplinary perspectives on hope* (pp. 3–23). Springer Open.

    Michener, R. T. (2020). Post-Kantian to postmodern considerations of (theological) hope. In S. C. van den Heuvel (Ed.), *Historical and multidisciplinary perspectives on hope* (pp. 77–97). Springer Open.

24. Cohen-Chen, S., Halperin, E., Crisp, R. J., & Gross, J. J. (2014). Hope in the Middle East: Malleability beliefs, hope, and the willingness to compromise for peace. *Social Psychological and Personality Science, 5*(1), 67–75.

    Sleat, M. (2013). Hope and disappointment in politics. *Contemporary Politics, 19*(2), 131–145.

25. Scioli, A. (2020). The psychology of hope: A diagnostic and prescriptive account. In S. C. van den Heuvel (Ed.), *Historical and multidisciplinary perspectives on hope* (pp. 137–163). Springer Open.

    Snyder, C. R. (Ed.). (2000). *Handbook of hope: Theory, measures, and applications*. Academic Press.

26. Cohen-Chen, S., Halperin, E., Crisp, R. J., & Gross, J. J. (2014). Hope in the Middle East: Malleability beliefs, hope, and the willingness to compromise for peace. *Social Psychological and Personality Science, 5*(1), 67–75.

    Petersen, A., & Wilkinson, I. (2015). Editorial introduction: The sociology of hope in contexts of health, medicine, and healthcare. *Health (London), 19*(2), 113–118.

27. Elliot, D. (2020). Hope in theology. In S. C. van den Heuvel (Ed.), *Historical and multidisciplinary perspectives on hope* (pp. 117–136). Springer Open.

    Wright, N. T. (2008). *Surprised by hope*. HarperOne.

28. Jarymowicz, M., & Bar-Tal, D. (2006). The dominance of fear over hope in the life of individuals and collectives. *European Journal of Social Psychology, 36*(3), 367–392.

29. Rustøen, T. (1995). Hope and quality of life, two central issues for cancer patients: A theoretical analysis. *Cancer Nursing, 18*(5), 355–361.

30. Olsman, E. (2020). Hope in health care: A synthesis of review studies. In S. C. van den Heuvel (Ed.), *Historical and multidisciplinary perspectives on hope* (pp. 197–214). Springer Open.

31. Duggleby, W., Hicks, D., Nekolaichuk, C., Holtslander, L., Williams, A., Chambers, T., & Eby, J. (2012). Hope, older adults, and chronic illness: A

metasynthesis of qualitative research. *Journal of Advanced Nursing, 68*(6), 1211–1223.

32. Karatepe, O. M. (2014). Hope, work engagement, and organizationally valued performance outcomes: An empirical study in the hotel industry. *Journal of Hospitality Marketing & Management, 23*(6), 678–698.

    Peterson, S. J., & Byron, K. (2007). Exploring the role of hope in job performance: Results from four studies. *Journal of Organizational Behavior, 28*(6), 785–803.

    Duggleby, W., Cooper, D., & Penz, K. (2009). Hope, self-efficacy, spiritual well-being and job satisfaction. *Journal of Advanced Nursing, 65*(11), 2376–2385.

33. Yotsidi, V., Pagoulatou, A., Kyriazos, T., & Stalikas, A. (2018). The role of hope in academic and work environments: An integrative literature review. *Psychology, 9*(3), 385–402.

34. Kortte, K. B., Stevenson, J. E., Hosey, M. M., Castillo, R., & Wegener, S. T. (2012). Hope predicts positive functional role outcomes in acute rehabilitation populations. *Rehabilitation Psychology, 57*(3), 248–255.

35. Bartholomew, T. T., Joy, E. E., & Gundel, B. E. (2021). Clients' hope for counseling as a redictor of outcome in psychotherapy. *The Counseling Psychologist, 49*(8), 1126–1146.

    Irving, L. M., Snyder, C. R., Cheavens, J., Gravel, L., Hanke, J., Hilberg, P., & Nelson, N. (2004). The relationships between hope and outcomes at the pretreatment, beginning, and later phases of psychotherapy. *Journal of Psychotherapy Integration, 14*(4), 419–443.

36. Bandura, A. (1982). Self-efficacy mechanism in human agency. *American Psychologist, 37*, 122–147.

    Hevey, D., Smith, M. l., & McGee, H. M. (1998). Self-efficacy and health behaviour: A review. *Irish Journal of Psychology, 19*(2–3), 248–273.

    O'Leary, A. (1985). Self-efficacy and health. *Behaviour Research and Therapy, 23*(4), 437–451.

37. Gravlee, G. S. (2020). Hope in ancient Greek philosophy. In S. C. van den Heuvel (Ed.), *Historical and multidisciplinary perspectives on hope* (pp. 3–23). Springer Open.

38. Pichalakkatt, B. J. (2013). Matter matters: The eschatology of matter. *European Journal of Science and Theology, 9*(3), 29–43.

    Teilhard de Chardin, P. (1964). *The future of man*. Doubleday.

39. Dr. Martin Luther King Jr. *Remaining awake through a great revolution*. Speech at the National Cathedral in Washington, D.C., March 31, 1968. An earlier

source of this quotation is the 19th-century Unitarian pastor and abolitionist Theodore Parker.

40. Luthans, F., Avey, J. B., Avolio, B. J., & Peterson, S. J. (2010). The development and resulting performance impact of positive psychological capital. *Human Resource Development Quarterly, 21*(1), 41–67.

41. Folkman, S. (2010). Stress, coping, and hope. *Psycho-Oncology, 19*(9), 901–908.

42. Olsman, E. (2020). Hope in health care: A synthesis of review studies. In S. C. van den Heuvel (Ed.), *Historical and multidisciplinary perspectives on hope* (pp. 197–214). Springer Open.

CHAPTER 2. Desire

1. Addams, J. (2019). *Twenty years at Hull-House.* IndoEuropean Publishing.
   www.nobelprize.org/prizes/peace/1931/addams/biographical
   www.womenshistory.org/education-resources/biographies/jane-addams
   https://en.wikipedia.org/wiki/Jane_Addams

2. Goddard, C., & Wierzbicka, A. (1994) *Semantic and lexical universals.* John Benjamins.

3. Rosenthal, R. (2002). The Pygmalion effect and its mediating mechanisms. In J. Aronson (Ed.), *Improving academic achievement: Impact of psychological factors on education* (pp. 25–36). Academic Press.
   Szumski, G., & Karwowski, M. (2019). Exploring the Pygmalion effect: The role of teacher expectations, academic self-concept, and class context in students' math achievement. *Contemporary Educational Psychology, 59.*

4. Eden, D. (1992). Leadership and expectations: Pygmalion effects and other self-fulfilling prophecies in organizations. *The Leadership Quarterly, 3*(4), 271–305.
   Inamori, T., & Analoui, F. (2010). Beyond Pygmalion effect: The role of managerial perception. *Journal of Management Development, 29*(4), 306–321.

5. Kierein, N. M., & Gold, M. A. (2000). Pygmalion in work organizations: A meta-analysis. *Journal of Organizational Behavior, 21*(8), 913–928.

6. Milona, M. (2020). Philosophy of hope. In S. C. van den Heuvel (Ed.), *Historical and multidisciplinary perspectives on hope* (pp. 99–116). Springer Open.

7. Wiles, R., Cott, C., & Gibson, B. E. (2008). Hope, expectations and recovery from illness: A narrative synthesis of qualitative research. *Journal of Advanced Nursing 64*(6), 564–573.

8. Milona, M. (2020). Philosophy of hope. In S. C. van den Heuvel (Ed.), *Historical and multidisciplinary perspectives on hope* (pp. 99–116). Springer Open.

9. van den Heuvel, S. C. (2020). *Historical and multidisciplinary perspectives on hope*. Springer Open.

10. Drahos, P. (2004). Trading in public hope. *Annals of the American Academy of Political and Social Science, 592*, 18–38.

11. Miller, W. R., & Rollnick, S. (2023). *Motivational interviewing: Helping people change and grow* (4th ed.). Guilford Press.

12. Rollnick, S. (1998). Readiness, importance, and confidence: Critical conditions of change in treatment. In W. R. Miller & N. Heather (Eds.), *Treating addictive behaviors* (2nd ed., pp. 49–60). Plenum Press.

    Miller, W. R., & Rollnick, S. (1991). *Motivational interviewing: Preparing people to change addictive behavior*. Guilford Press.

13. Snyder, C. R. (1994). *The psychology of hope*. Free Press.

    Snyder, C. R. (Ed.). (2000). *Handbook of hope: Theory, measures, and applications*. Academic Press.

14. Snyder, C. R., Harris, C., Anderson, J. R., Holleran, S. A., Irving, L. M., Sigmon, S. T., . . . Harney, P. (1991). The will and the ways: Development and validation of an individual-differences measure of hope. *Journal of Personality and Social Psychology, 60*(4), 570–585.

15. Leshem, O. A., & Halperin, E. (2020). Hope during conflict. In S. C. van den Heuvel (Ed.), *Historical and multidisciplinary perspectives on hope* (pp. 179–196). Springer Open.

16. Bernardo, A. B. I. (2010). Extending hope theory: Internal and external locus of trait hope. *Personality and Individual Differences, 49*(8), 944–949.

    Gallagher, M. W., & Lopez, S. J. (2009). Positive expectancies and mental health: Identifying the unique contributions of hope and optimism. *Journal of Positive Psychology, 4*(6), 548–556.

17. Kortte, K. B., Stevenson, J. E., Hosey, M. M., Castillo, R., & Wegener, S. T. (2012). Hope predicts positive functional role outcomes in acute rehabilitation populations. *Rehabilitation Psychology, 57*(3), 248–255.

18. Bandura, A. (1997). *Self-efficacy: The exercise of control*. Freeman.

19. Gollwitzer, P. M. (1999). Implementation intentions: Strong effects of simple plans. *American Psychologist, 54*(7), 493–503.

20. Pinsent, A. (2020). Hope as a virtue in the Middle Ages. In S. C. van den Heuvel (Ed.), *Historical and multidisciplinary perspectives on hope* (pp. 47–60). Springer Open.

21. Thurman, H. (1996). *Jesus and the disinherited*. Beacon Press.

22. Elliott, R., Bohart, A. C., Watson, J. C., & Greenberg, L. S. (2011). Empathy. *Psychotherapy, 48*(1), 43–49.

    Moyers, T. B., & Miller, W. R. (2013). Is low therapist empathy toxic? *Psychology of Addictive Behaviors, 27*(3), 878–884.

23. Kylmä, J., Duggleby, W., Cooper, D., & Molander, G. (2009). Hope in palliative care: An integrative review. *Palliative and Supportive Care, 7*(3), 365–377.

24. Leake, G. J., & King, A. S. (1977). Effect of counselor expectations on alcoholic recovery. *Alcohol Health & Research World, 1*(3), 16–22.

25. Downey, G., Freitas, A. L., Michaelis, B., & Khouri, H. (1998). The self-fulfilling prophecy in close relationships: Rejection sensitivity and rejection by romantic partners. *Journal of Personality and Social Psychology, 75*(2), 545–560.

26. This point was poignantly made by Mark Twain in his short story "The War Prayer," which, by his request, was unpublished until after his death. Twain, M. (2015). *The war prayer*. Rough Draft Printing.

27. Cannon, W. B. (1942). "Voodoo" death. *American Anthropologist, 44*(2), 169–181.

28. Sternberg, E. M. (2002). Walter B. Cannon and "voodoo death": A perspective from 60 years on. *American Journal of Public Health, 92*(10), 1564–1566.

29. Merton, R. K. (1948). The self-fulfilling prophecy. *Antioch Review, 8*(2), 193–210.

30. Jussim, L. (1986). Self-fulfilling prophecies: A theoretical and integrative review. *Psychological Review, 93*(4), 429–445.

31. Snyder, M., & Swann, W. B., Jr. (1978). Behavioral confirmation in social interaction: From social perception to social reality. *Journal of Experimental Social Psychology, 14*, 148–162.

32. Chen, M., & Bargh, J. A. (1997). Nonconscious behavioral confirmation processes: The self-fulfilling consequences of automatic stereotype activation. *Journal of Experimental Social Psychology, 33*(5), 541–560.

33. Rosenhan, D. L. (1973). On being sane in insane places. *Science, 179*, 250–258.

34. Becker, K. J., Baxter, A. B., Cohen, W. A., Bybee, H. M., Tirschwell, D. L., Newell, D. W., . . . Longstreth, W. T. (2001). Withdrawal of support in intracerebral hemorrhage may lead to self-fulfilling prophecies. *Neurology, 56*(6), 766–772.

35. Haley, A., & Malcolm X. (1964). *The autobiography of Malcolm X as told to Alex Haley* (pp. 38–39). Ballantine.

36. Nowinski, J. (2004). Evil by default: The origins of dark visions. *Journal of Clinical Psychology: In Session, 60*, 519–530.

37. A classic example is dramatized in the Frank Capra film *It's a Wonderful Life*.

38. Kahneman, D. (2011). *Thinking, fast and slow*. Farrar, Straus and Giroux.
    Nickerson, R. S. (1998). Confirmation bias: A ubiquitous phenomenon in many guises. *Review of General Psychology, 2*(2), 175–220.

39. Simons, D. J., & Chabris, C. F. (1999). Gorillas in our midst: Sustained inattentional blindness for dynamic events. *Perception, 28*(9), 1059–1074.

40. Carver, S. C., & White, T. L. (1994). Behavioral inhibition, behavioral activation, and affective responses to impending reward and punishment: The BIS/BAS scales. *Journal of Personality and Social Psychology, 67*, 319–333.
    Gray, J. A. (1990). Brain systems that mediate both emotion and cognition. *Cognition and Emotion, 4*, 269–288.

41. McSorley, E., & Morriss, J. (2017). What you see is what you want to see: Motivationally relevant stimuli can interrupt current resource allocation. *Cognition and Emotion, 31*(1), 168–174.

42. Strachman, A., & Gable, S. L. (2006). What you want (and do not want) affects what you see (and do not see): Avoidance social goals and social events. *Personality and Social Psychology Bulletin, 32*(11), 1446–1458.

43. Nikitin, J., & Freund, A. M. (2015). What you want to avoid is what you see: Social avoidance motivation affects the interpretation of emotional faces. *Motivation and Emotion, 39*(3), 384–391.

44. Balcetis, E., & Dunning, D. (2006). See what you want to see: Motivational influences on visual perception. *Journal of Personality and Social Psychology, 91*(4), 612–625.

45. Blöser, C. (2020). Enlightenment views of hope. In S. C. van den Heuvel (Ed.), *Historical and multidisciplinary perspectives on hope* (pp. 61–76). Springer Open.

46. Over the years our research group at the University of New Mexico developed several effective earlier interventions, including motivational interviewing, behavioral self-control training, and the community reinforcement and family training (CRAFT) method that have touched many lives.

47. McLellan, A. T., Koob, G. F., & Volkow, N. D. (2022). Pre-addiction—A missing concept for treating substance use disorders. *JAMA Psychiatry, 79*(8), 749–751.

48. Yahne, C. E., & Miller, W. R. (1999). Evoking hope. In W. R. Miller (Ed.), *Integrating spirituality into treatment: Resources for practitioners* (pp. 217–233). American Psychological Association.

49. Miller, W. R., & Rollnick, S. (2023). *Motivational interviewing: Helping people change and grow* (4th ed.). Guilford Press.

50. Miller, W. R., & Moyers, T. B. (2021). *Effective psychotherapists: Clinical skills that improve client outcomes.* Guilford Press.

    Orlinsky, D. E., Grawe, K., & Parks, B. K. (1994). Process and outcome in psychotherapy: Noch einmal. In A. E. Bergin & S. L. Garfield (Eds.), *Handbook of psychotherapy and behavior change* (pp. 270–376). Wiley.

51. Snyder, C. R. (1994). *The psychology of hope.* Free Press.

52. Langer, E. J. (1989). *Mindfulness.* Addison-Wesley.

53. LaMotte, D. (2014). *Worldchanging 101: Challenging the myth of powerlessness.* Dryad.

    Macy, J., & Johnstone, C. (2022). *Active hope: How to face the mess we're in with unexpected resilience & creative power* (rev. ed.). New World Library.

CHAPTER 3. Probability

1. Jonathan Capehart on *PBS NewsHour*, June 3, 2023.

2. The classic terms for these coping styles are repression (avoid and forget) versus sensitization (approach and explore). Byrne, D. (1964). Repression–sensitization as a dimension of personality. *Progress in Experimental Personality Research, 72,* 169–220.

    Hock, M., & Kohlmann, C. W. (2020). Repression-sensitization. In *Encyclopedia of personality and individual differences* (pp. 4428–4432). Springer International.

3. I think here of the fox in Chapter 21 of Antoine de Saint-Exupery's classic story *The Little Prince.*

4. Bargh, J. A., & Chartrand, T. L. (1999). The unbearable automaticity of being. *American Psychologist, 54,* 462–479.

5. Monahan, J. (1984). The prediction of violent behavior. *American Journal of Psychiatry, 141*(1), 10–15.

    Edens, J. F., Buffington-Vollum, J. K., Keilen, A., Roskamp, P., & Anthony, C. (2005). Predictions of future dangerousness in capital murder trials: Is it time to "disinvent the wheel?" *Law and Human Behavior 29*(1), 55–86.

6. Morris, N., & Miller, M. (1985). Predictions of dangerousness. *Crime and Justice, 6,* 1–50.

7. C'de Baca, J., Miller, W. R., & Laham, S. (2001). A multiple risk factor approach for predicting DWI recidivism. *Journal of Substance Abuse Treatment, 21,* 207–215.

8. Wiggins, J. S. (1973). *Personality and prediction: Principles of personality assessment*. Addison-Wesley.

9. Goldberg, L. R. (1970). Man versus model of man: A rationale plus evidence for a method of improving clinical inferences. *Psychological Bulletin, 73,* 422–432.

10. Morris, N., & Miller, M. (1985). Predictions of dangerousness. *Crime and Justice, 6,* 1–50.

11. Price, D. D., Riley, J., & Barrell, J. J. (2001). Are lived choices based on emotional processes? *Cognition and Emotion, 15*(3), 365–379.

12. Grant, A. (2021). *Think again: The power of knowing what you don't know.* Viking Press.

Kahneman, D. (2011). *Thinking, fast and slow.* Farrar, Straus and Giroux.

Tversky, A., & Kahneman, D. (1974). Judgment under uncertainty: Heuristics and biases. *Science, 185*(4157), 1124–1131.

13. Gladwell, M. (2007). *Blink: The power of thinking without thinking.* Little, Brown & Company.

14. Forgas, J. P., & Laham, S. M. (2017). Halo effects. In R. F. Pohl (Ed.), *Cognitive illusions: Intriguing phenomena in thinking, judgment and memory* (2nd ed., pp. 276–290). Routledge.

15. Mayer, J. D., Gaschke, Y. N., Braverman, D. L., & Evans, T. W. (1992). Mood-congruent judgment is a general effect. *Journal of Personality and Social Psychology, 63*(1), 119–132.

Tversky, A., & Kahneman, D. (1973). Availability: A heuristic for judging frequency and probability. *Cognitive Psychology, 5*(2), 207–232.

16. Massey, C., Simmons, J. P., & Armor, D. A. (2011). Hope over experience: Desirability and the persistence of optimism. *Psychological Science, 22*(2), 274–281.

17. Blanchette, I., & Richards, A. (2010). The influence of affect on higher level cognition: A review of research on interpretation, judgement, decision making and reasoning. *Cognition and Emotion 24*(4), 561–595.

18. Amrhein, P. C. (1992). The comprehension of quasi-performance verbs in verbal commitments: New evidence for componential theories of lexical meaning. *Journal of Memory and Language, 31,* 756–784.

19. Davidson, L., & McGlashan, T. H. (1997). The varied outcomes of schizophrenia. *Canadian Journal of Psychiatry, 42*(1), 34–43.

Miller, W. R., Walters, S. T., & Bennett, M. E. (2001). How effective is alcoholism treatment in the United States? *Journal of Studies on Alcohol, 62,* 211–220.

20. Kirkpatrick, H., Landeen, J., Woodside, H., & Byrne, C. (2001). How people

with schizophrenia build their hope. *Journal of Psychosocial Nursing and Mental Health Services 39*(1), 46–55.

Leake, G. J., & King, A. S. (1977). Effect of counselor expectations on alcoholic recovery. *Alcohol Health & Research World, 1*(3), 16–22.

21. Miller, W. R. (2015). Retire the concept of "relapse." *Substance Use & Misuse, 50*(8–9), 976–977.

22. Miller, W. R., Walters, S. T., & Bennett, M. E. (2001). How effective is alcoholism treatment in the United States? *Journal of Studies on Alcohol, 62*, 211–220.

23. To assist treatment professionals I published successive reviews of the large body of clinical trials on treating addictions. For example: Miller, W. R., & Wilbourne, P. L. (2002). Mesa Grande: A methodological analysis of clinical trials of treatment for alcohol use disorders. *Addiction, 97*(3), 265–277.

    Miller, W. R., Forcehimes, A. A., & Zweben, A. (2019). *Treating addiction: A guide for professionals* (2nd ed.). Guilford Press.

24. This very good question was once posed by author Mitch Albom.

25. Petersen, A., Tanner, C., & Munsie, M. (2015). Between hope and evidence: How community advisors demarcate the boundary between legitimate and illegitimate stem cell treatments. *Health (London), 19*(2), 188–206.

26. Kübler-Ross, E., & Kessler, D. (2014). *On grief and grieving: Finding the meaning of grief through the five stages of loss*. Scribner.

    Kübler-Ross, E. (2014). *On death and dying: What the dying have to teach doctors, nurses, clergy and their own families* (50th anniversary edition). Scribner.

27. Chen, H., Komaromy, C., & Valentine, C. (2015). From hope to hope: The experience of older Chinese people with advanced cancer. *Health (London), 19*(2), 154–171.

28. Tillich, P. (1965). The right to hope. *University of Chicago Magazine, 58*(2), 16–21.

29. Gravlee, G. S. (2020). Hope in ancient Greek philosophy. In S. C. van den Heuvel (Ed.), *Historical and multidisciplinary perspectives on hope* (pp. 3–23). Springer Open.

30. Ashcraft, T. O., & McGearhart, S. (2003). *Red sky in mourning: A true story of love, loss, and survival at sea*. Hachette Books.

31. Franklin, J. (2015). *438 days: An extraordinary true story of survival at sea*. Atria Books.

32. Rotter, J. B. (1966). Generalized expectancies for internal versus external control of reinforcement. *Psychological Monographs: General and Applied, 80*(1, Whole No. 609), 1–28.

33. Antwi-Boasiako, B. A. (2017). It's beyond my control: The effect of locus of control orientation on disaster insurance adoption. *International Journal of Disaster Risk Reduction, 22,* 297–303.

Baumann, D. D., & Sims, J. H. (1978). Flood insurance: Some determinants of adoption. *Economic Geography, 54*(3), 189–196.

34. Giuliani, M., Ichino, A., Bonomi, A., Martoni, R., Cammino, S., & Gorini, A. (2021). Who is willing to get vaccinated? A study into the psychological, socio-demographic, and cultural determinants of COVID-19 vaccination intentions. *Vaccines, 9*(8), 810–831.

35. Sims, J. H., & Baumann, D. D. (1972). The tornado threat: Coping styles of the North and South. *Science, 176*(4042), 1386–1392.

36. McCarty, J. A., & Shrum, L. J. (2001). The influence of individualism, collectivism, and locus of control on environmental beliefs and behavior. *Journal of Public Policy and Marketing, 20*(1), 93–104.

37. McNairn, H. E., & Mitchell, B. (1992). Locus of control and farmer orientation: Effects on conservation adoption. *Journal of Agricultural and Environmental Ethics, 5*(1), 87–101.

38. Kalamas, M., Cleveland, M., & Laroche, M. (2014). Pro-environmental behaviors for thee but not for me: Green giants, green gods, and external environmental locus of control. *Journal of Business Research, 67*(2), 12–22.

Mostafa, M. M. (2016). Post-materialism, religiosity, political orientation, locus of control and concern for global warming: A multilevel analysis across 40 nations. *Social Indicators Research, 128*(3), 1273–1298.

39. Reimann, M., Nenkov, G. Y., MacInnis, D., & Morrin, M. (2014). The role of hope in financial risk seeking. *Journal of Experimental Psychology: Applied, 20*(4), 349–364.

40. Brooks, M. J., Marshal, M. P., McCauley, H. L., Douaihy, A., & Miller, E. (2016). The relationship between hope and adolescent likelihood to endorse substance use behaviors in a sample of marginalized youth. *Substance Use and Misuse, 51*(13), 1815–1819.

41. Rand, K. L., & Cheavens, J. S. (2009). Hope theory. In S. J. Lopez & C. R. Snyder (Eds.), *Oxford handbook of positive psychology* (2nd ed., pp. 323–334). Oxford University Press.

42. Jones, R. A. (1981). *Self-fulfilling prophecies: Social, psychological, and physiological effects of expectancies.* Psychology Press.

43. Curry, L. A., Snyder, C. R., Cook, D. L., Ruby, B. C., & Rehm, M. (1997). Role of hope in academic and sport achievement. *Journal of Personality and Social Psychology, 73*(6), 1257–1267.

Snyder, C. R. (1994). *The psychology of hope.* Free Press.

44. Miller, W. R. (2017). *Lovingkindness: Realizing and practicing your true self.* Cascade Books.

45. Moltmann, J. (1993). *Theology of hope.* Fortress Press.

CHAPTER 4. Possibility

1. Source: *https://en.wikipedia.org/wiki/Anne_Sullivan;* accessed 7/30/22.

2. Moltmann, J. (1993). *Theology of hope.* Fortress Press.

3. This quotation is not from the original Cervantes novel, but is voiced by Don Quixote in the play *The Man of la Mancha.*

4. *www.census.gov/library/stories/2023/01/volunteering-and-civic-life-in-america. html#:~:text=Related%20Statistics&text=The%202021%20Volunteering%20 in%20America,was%20estimated%20at%20%24122.9B.&text=The%20 U.S.%20Census%20Bureau%20and%20AmeriCorps%20announced%20 the%20release%20of,(CEV)%20Supplement%20Microdata%20File.*

5. Kim, E. S., Whillans, A. V., Lee, M. T., Chen, Y., & VanderWeele, T. J. (2020). Volunteering and subsequent health and well-being in older adults: An outcome-wide longitudinal approach. *American Journal of Preventive Medicine, 59*(2), 176–186.

6. Rohr, R. (2023, October 11). *True realism.* Daily meditation from the Center for Action and Contemplation, Albuquerque, New Mexico.

7. Murray, S. L., Holmes, J. G., & Griffin, D. W. (1996). The self-fulfilling nature of positive illusions in romantic relationships: Love is not blind, but prescient. *Journal of Personality and Social Psychology, 71*(6), 1155–1180.

8. 60 years later I still remember the chorus: Tinniat, tinniat tintinnabulum. Labimur in glacie post mulum curtum.

9. Morgen, morgen, lacht uns wieder das Glück.

10. Thurman, H. (1976). *Jesus and the disinherited.* Beacon Press.

11. John 8:2–11. J. B. Phillips translation.

12. Quoted with permission from Miller, W. R., Forcehimes, A. A., & Zweben, A. (2019). *Treating addiction: A guide for professionals* (2nd ed.). Guilford Press.

13. Our research group noticed this in a large study treating alcohol problems in which people given placebo medication showed larger reductions in drinking, compared with those given no pills at all.

Anton, R. F., O'Malley, S. S., Ciraulo, D. A., Cisler, R. A., Couper, D., Donovan, D. M., . . . Zweben, A. (2006). Combined pharmacotherapies and behavioral interventions for alcohol dependence: The COMBINE study, a randomized controlled trial. *Journal of the American Medical Association, 295*(17), 2003–2017.

Weiss, R. D., LoCastro, J., Swift, R., Zweben, A., Miller, W. R., Longabaugh, R., & Hosking, J. D. (2005). The use of a "psychotherapy with no pills" treatment condition as part of a combined pharmacotherapy-psychotherapy research study of alcohol dependence. *Journal of Studies on Alcohol, Suppl. No. 15*, 43–49.

14. Price, D. D., Finniss, D. G., & Benedetti, F. (2008). A comprehensive review of the placebo effect: Recent advances and current thought. *Annual Review of Psychology, 59*(1), 565–590.

Colagiuri, B., Schenk, L. A., Kessler, M. D., Dorsey, S. G., & Colloca, L. (2015). The placebo effect: From concepts to genes. *Neuroscience, 307,* 171–190.

15. Vase, L., Riley, J. L., & Price, D. D. (2002). A comparison of placebo effects in clinical analgesic trials versus studies of placebo analgesia. *Pain, 99*(3), 443–452.

16. Marlatt, G. A., Demming, B., & Reid, J. B. (1973). Loss of control drinking in alcoholics: An experimental analogue. *Journal of Abnormal Psychology, 81,* 223–241.

17. Hull, J. G., & Bond, C. F. J. (1986). Social and behavioral consequences of alcohol consumption and expectancy: A meta-analysis. *Psychological Bulletin, 99*(3), 347–360.

18. Kaptchuk, T. J. (2018). Open-label placebo: Reflections on a research agenda. *Perspectives in Biology and Medicine, 61*(3), 311–334.

19. Kaptchuk, T. J. (2018). Open-label placebo: Reflections on a research agenda. *Perspectives in Biology and Medicine, 61*(3), 313, 321–322 (italics added).

20. Franklin, B. (1785). *Report of Dr. Benjamin Franklin, and other commissioners, charged by the King of France, with the examination of the animal magnetism, as now practised at Paris.* J. Johnson.

21. Franklin, B. (1785). *Report of Dr. Benjamin Franklin, and other commissioners, charged by the King of France, with the examination of the animal magnetism, as now practised at Paris.* J. Johnson. Quotations from pp. 100 and 102.

22. Schmidt, M. M., & Miller, W. R. (1983). Amount of therapist contact and outcome in a multidimensional depression treatment program. *Acta Psychiatrica Scandinavica, 67*(5), 319–332.

23. Miller, W. R., & Moyers, T. B. (2021). *Effective psychotherapists: Clinical skills that improve client outcomes.* Guilford Press.

24. Franklin, B. (1785). *Report of Dr. Benjamin Franklin, and other commissioners, charged by the King of France, with the examination of the animal magnetism, as now practised at Paris.* J. Johnson. Quotation from p. xii.

25. Thurman, H. (1976). *Jesus and the disinherited* (p. 36). Beacon Press.

26. Brown, P., de Graaf, S., & Hillen, M. (2015). The inherent tensions and ambiguities of hope: Towards a post-formal analysis of experiences of advanced-cancer patients. *Health (London), 19*(2), 207–225.

   Folkman, S. (2010). Stress, coping, and hope. *Psycho-Oncology, 19*(9), 901–908.

27. Myers, I. B., & Myers, P. B. (2010). *Gifts differing: Understanding personality type* (rev. ed.). Davies-Black.

   Myers, I. B., McCaulley, M. H., Quenk, N. L., & Hammer, A. L. (1998). *MBTI manual: A guide to the development and use of the Myers-Briggs Type Indicator* (3rd ed.). Consulting Psychologists Press.

28. Kiersey, D. (2006). *Please understand me II: Temperament, character, intelligence*. Prometheus Nemesis Book Company.

29. Zehr, H. (2014). *The little book of restorative justice* (rev. ed.). Good Books.

30. Bandura, A. (1997). *Self-efficacy: The exercise of control*. Freeman.

31. Cohen-Chen, S., Halperin, E., Crisp, R. J., & Gross, J. J. (2014). Hope in the Middle East: Malleability beliefs, hope, and the willingness to compromise for peace. *Social Psychological and Personality Science, 5*(1), 67–75.

32. The escape route that was offered actually varied across experiments, but a push button is one illustrative example.

33. Gatchel, R. J. (1980). Perceived control: A review and evaluation of therapeutic implications. In A. Baum & J. E. Singer (Eds.), *Advances in environmental psychology* (Vol. 2: Applications of personal control, pp. 1–24). Erlbaum.

   Glass, D. C., Singer, J. E., Leonard, H. S., Krantz, D., Cohen, S., & Cummings, H. (1973). Perceived control of aversive stimulation and the reduction of stress responses. *Journal of Personality, 41*(4), 577–595.

34. Talley, J. E. (1992). *The predictors of successful very brief psychotherapy: A study of differences by gender, age, and treatment variables*. Charles C Thomas.

35. Miller, W. R., Benefield, R. G., & Tonigan, J. S. (1993). Enhancing motivation for change in problem drinking: A controlled comparison of two therapist styles. *Journal of Consulting and Clinical Psychology, 61*, 455–461.

36. Harris, K. B., & Miller, W. R. (1990). Behavioral self-control training for problem drinkers: Components of efficacy. *Psychology of Addictive Behaviors, 4*, 82–90.

37. Miller, W. R., & Muñoz, R. F. (2013). *Controlling your drinking* (2nd ed.). Guilford Press.

38. Miller, W. R. (2015). No more waiting lists! *Substance Use and Misuse, 50*(8–9), 1169–1170.

39. Snyder, C. R. (2002). Hope theory; Rainbows in the mind. *Psychological Inquiry 13*(4), 249–275.

40. Snyder, C. R., Irving, L. M., & Anderson, J. R. (1991). Hope and health. In C. R. Snyder & D. R. Forsyth (Eds.), *Handbook of social and clinical psychology: The health perspective* (pp. 285–305). Pergamon Press.

    Snyder, C. R., Lapointe, A. B., Crowson, J. J., Jr., & Early, S. (1998). Preferences of high- and low-hope people for self-referential input. *Cognition and Emotion, 12*, 807–823.

    Griggs, S., & Walker, R. K. (2016). The role of hope for adolescents with a chronic illness: An integrative review. *Journal of Pediatric Nursing, 31*(4), 404–421.

41. Folkman, S. (2010). Stress, coping, and hope. *Psycho-Oncology, 19*(9), 901–908.

    Petersen, A., & Wilkinson, I. (2015). Editorial introduction: The sociology of hope in contexts of health, medicine, and healthcare. *Health (London), 19*(2), 113–118.

42. I thank Richard Rohr for this insight, that people see things not only as they are, but also as *they* are.

CHAPTER 5. Optimism: High Hopes

1. Starr, M. (2013). *The showings of Julian of Norwich: A new translation*. Hampton Roads. The saint's actual name is unknown. She is called Julian or Juliana of Norwich after the Church of St. Julian in Norwich, England, to which her anchor-hold cell was attached, and in which she lived for four decades.

2. Reichard, R. J., Avey, J. B., Lopez, S., & Dollwet, M. (2013). Having the will and finding the way: A review and meta-analysis of hope at work. *Journal of Positive Psychology, 8*(4), 292–304.

3. Luthans, F., Avey, J. B., Avolio, B. J., & Peterson, S. J. (2010). The development and resulting performance impact of positive psychological capital. *Human Resource Development Quarterly, 21*(1), 41–67.

4. Scheier, M. F., Carver, C. S., & Bridges, M. W. (1994). Distinguishing optimism from neuroticism (and trait anxiety, self-mastery, and self-esteem): A reevaluation of the Life Orientation Test. *Journal of Personality and Social Psychology, 67*(6), 1063–1078.

5. Armor, D. A., & Taylor, S. E. (1998). Situated optimism: Specific outcome expectancies and self-regulation. In M. P. Zanna (Ed.), *Advances in experimental social psychology* (Vol. 30, pp. 309–379). Academic Press.

6. Bailey, T. C., Eng, W., Frisch, M. B., & Snyder, C. R. (2007). Hope and optimism as related to life satisfaction. *Journal of Positive Psychology, 2*(3), 168–175.

Bandura, A. (1997). *Self-efficacy: The exercise of control.* Freeman.

Bandura, A. (2008). An agentic perspective on positive psychology. In S. J. Lopez (Ed.), *Positive psychology: Exploring the best in people* (Vol. 1, pp. 167–196). Greenwood.

Luthans, F., & Jensen, S. M. (2002). Hope: A new positive strength for human resource development. *Human Resource Development Review, 1*(3), 304–322.

Luthans, F., Vogelgesang, G. R., & Lester, P. B. (2006). Developing the psychological capital of resiliency. *Human Resource Development Review, 5,* 25–44.

7. Masten, A. S., & Reed, M.-G. J. (2002). Resilience in development. In C. R. Snyder & S. J. Lopez (Eds.), *Handbook of positive psychology* (pp. 74–88). Oxford University Press.

8. Peterson, C., & Seligman, M. E. P. (2004). Hope. In *Character strengths and virtues: A handbook and classification.* Oxford University Press. Quotation from p. 572.

9. *https://ufw.org/history-si-se-puede*, downloaded March 29, 2023.

10. Luthans, F., Avey, J. B., Avolio, B. J., & Peterson, S. J. (2010). The development and resulting performance impact of positive psychological capital. *Human Resource Development Quarterly, 21*(1), 41–67.

11. From a 1948 short story "Narapoia" by Alan Nelson. Kopp, S. B. (1978). Narapoia. *Journal of Contemporary Psychotherapy, 10,* 46–47.

12. Peterson, C., & Seligman, M. E. P. (2004). *Character strengths and virtues: A handbook and classification.* Oxford University Press. Quotation from p. 572.

13. Pleeging, E., Burger, M., & van Exel, J. (2021). The relations between hope and subjective well-being: A literature overview and empirical analysis. *Applied Research in Quality of Life, 16,* 1019–1041.

14. Brissette, I., Scheier, M. F., & Carver, C. S. (2002). The role of optimism in social network development, coping, and psychological adjustment during a life transition. *Journal of Personality and Social Psychology, 82*(1), 102–111.

Falavarjani, M. F., & Yeh, C. J. (2019). Optimism and distress tolerance in the social adjustment of nurses: Examining resilience as a mediator and gender as a moderator. *Journal of Research in Nursing, 24*(7), 500–512.

Tetzner, J., & Becker, M. (2015). How being an optimist makes a difference: The protective role of optimism in adolescents' adjustment to parental separation. *Social Psychological and Personality Science, 6*(3), 325–333.

15. Kwon, P. (2002). Hope, defense mechanisms, and adjustment: Implications for false hope and defensive hopelessness. *Journal of Personality, 70*(2), 207–231.

16. Rasmussen, H. N., Scheier, M. F., & Greenhouse, J. B. (2009). Optimism and physical health: A meta-analytic review. *Annals of Behavioral Medicine 37*(3), 239–256.

17. Southerland, J. L., Slawson, D. L., Pack, R., Sörensen, S., Lyness, J. M., & Hirsch, J. K. (2016). Trait hope and preparation for future care needs among older adult primary care patients. *Clinical Gerontologist, 39*(2), 117–126.

18. Scheier, M. F., Carver, C. S., & Bridges, M. W. (1994). Distinguishing optimism from neuroticism (and trait anxiety, self-mastery, and self-esteem): A reevaluation of the Life Orientation Test. *Journal of Personality and Social Psychology, 67*(6), 1063–1078.

19. Giltay, E. J., Geleijnse, J. M., Zitman, F. G., Hoekstra, T., & Schouten, E. G. (2004). Dispositional optimism and all-cause and cardiovascular mortality in a prospective cohort of elderly Dutch men and women. *Archives of General Psychiatry, 61*(11), 1126–1135.

20. Schiavon, C. C., Marchetti, E., Gurgel, L. G., Busnello, F. M., & Reppold, C. T. (2017). Optimism and hope in chronic disease: A systematic review. *Frontiers in Psychology, 7.*

21. Kwon, P. (2002). Hope, defense mechanisms, and adjustment: Implications for false hope and defensive hopelessness. *Journal of Personality, 70*(2), 207–231.

22. Pleeging, E., Burger, M., & van Exel, J. (2021). The relations between hope and subjective well-being: A literature overview and empirical analysis. *Applied Research in Quality of Life, 16*, 1019–1041.

23. Reichard, R. J., Avey, J. B., Lopez, S., & Dollwet, M. (2013). Having the will and finding the way: A review and meta-analysis of hope at work. *Journal of Positive Psychology, 8*(4), 292–304.

24. Peterson, C., & Seligman, M. E. P. (2004). Hope. In *Character strengths and virtues: A handbook and classification* (pp. 569–582). Oxford University Press.

25. Stinson, D. A., Cameron, J. J., Wood, J. V., Gaucher, D., & Holmes, J. G. (2009). Deconstructing the "reign of error": Interpersonal warmth explains the self-fulfilling prophecy of anticipated acceptance. *Personality and Social Psychology Bulletin, 35*(9), 1165–1178.

26. Dimino, K., Horan, K. M., & Stephenson, C. (2020). Leading our frontline HEROES through times of crisis with a sense of hope, efficacy, resilience, and optimism. *Nurse Leader, 18*(6), 592–596.
    Smith, P. A., & Hoy, W. K. (2007). Academic optimism and student achievement in urban elementary schools. *Journal of Educational Administration, 45*(5), 556–568.

27. Johnson, D. D. P., & Fowler, J. H. (2011). The evolution of overconfidence. *Nature, 477*, 317–320.

28. Klein, C. T. F., & Helweg-Larsen, M. (2002). Perceived control and the optimistic bias: A meta-analytic review. *Psychology & Health, 17*(4), 437–446.

    Pietruska, K., & Armony, J. L. (2013). Differential effects of trait anger on optimism and risk behaviour. *Cognition and Emotion, 27*(2), 318–325.

29. Chambers, J. R., & Windschitl, P. D. (2004). Biases in social comparative judgments: The role of nonmotivated factors in above-average and comparative-optimism effects. *Psychological Bulletin, 130*(5), 813–838.

30. Lillian optimistically wanted to tell her story with the hope that it might encourage others, so we wrote a joint father–daughter account through alternating chapters of the experience of adopting and being adopted as an older child.

    Miller, W. R., & Homer, L. K. (2016). *Portals: Two lives intertwined by adoption.* Wipf & Stock.

31. Pleeging, E., Burger, M., & van Exel, J. (2021). The relations between hope and subjective well-being: A literature overview and empirical analysis. *Applied Research in Quality of Life, 16,* 1019–1041.

    Munro, G. D., & Stansbury, J. A. (2009). The dark side of self-affirmation: Confirmation bias and illusory correlation in response to threatening information. *Personality and Social Psychology Bulletin, 35*(9), 1143–1153.

32. Petersen, L. R., Clark, M. M., Novotny, P., Kung, S., Sloan, J. A., Patten, C. A., . . . Colligan, R. C. (2008). Relationship of optimism–pessimism and health-related quality of life in breast cancer survivors. *Journal of Psychosocial Oncology, 26*(4), 15–32.

    Plomin, R., Scheier, M. F., Bergeman, C. S., Pedersen, N. L., Nesselroade, J. R., & McClearn, G. E. (1992). Optimism, pessimism and mental health: A twin/adoption analysis. *Personality and Individual Differences, 13*(8), 921–930.

33. Peterson, C., Seligman, M. E., & Vaillant, G. E. (1988). Pessimistic explanatory style is a risk factor for physical illness: A thirty-five-year longitudinal study. *Journal of Personality and Social Psychology, 55*(1), 23–27.

34. Bem, S. L. (1974). The measurement of psychological androgyny. *Journal of Consulting and Clinical Psychology, 42*(2), 155–162.

35. Scheier, M. F., Swanson, J. D., Barlow, M. A., Greenhouse, J. B., Wrosch, C., & Tindle, H. A. (2021). Optimism versus pessimism as predictors of physical health: A comprehensive reanalysis of dispositional optimism research. *American Psychologist, 76*(3), 529–548.

36. Stinson, D. A., Cameron, J. J., Wood, J. V., Gaucher, D., & Holmes, J. G. (2009). Deconstructing the "reign of error": Interpersonal warmth explains the self-fulfilling prophecy of anticipated acceptance. *Personality and Social Psychology Bulletin, 35*(9), 1165–1178.

37. Peterson, C., Maier, S. F., & Seligman, M. E. P. (1995). *Learned helplessness: A theory for the age of personal control*. Oxford University Press.

38. Miller, W. R., & Seligman, M. E. P. (1975). Depression and learned helplessness in man. *Journal of Abnormal Psychology, 84*(3), 228–238.

39. Hirito, D. S. (1974). Locus of control and learned helplessness. *Journal of Experimental Psychology, 102*(2), 187–193.

40. Maier, S. F., & Seligman, M. E. (2016). Learned helplessness at fifty: Insights from neuroscience. *Psychological Review, 123*(4), 349–367.

Dimidjian, S., Barrera, M., Jr., Martell, C., Muñoz, R. F., & Lewinsohn, P. M. (2011). The origins and current status of behavioral activation treatments for depression. *Annual Review of Clinical Psychology, 7*, 1–38.

Lewinsohn, P. M., Muñoz, R. F., Youngren, M. A., & Zeiss, A. M. (1992). *Control your depression* (rev. ed.). Fireside.

Muñoz, R. F., Le, H.-N., Clarke, G. N., Barrera, A. Z., & Torres, L. D. (2009). Preventing first onset and recurrence of major depressive episodes. In I. H. Gotlib & C. L. Hammen (Eds.), *Handbook of depression* (2nd ed., pp. 533–553). Guilford Press.

41. Zimmerman, M. A. (1990). Toward a theory of learned hopefulness: A structural model analysis of participation and empowerment. *Journal of Research in Personality, 24*, 71–86.

Seligman, M. E. P. (2006). *Learned optimism: How to change your mind and your life*. Vintage Books.

Tomasulo, D. (2020). *Learned hopefulness: The power of positivity to overcome depression*. New Harbinger.

42. Hammond, V. L., Watson, P. J., O'Leary, B. J., & Cothran, D. L. (2009). Preliminary assessment of Apache hopefulness: Relationships with hopelessness and with collective as well as personal self-esteem. *American Indian and Alaska Native Mental Health Research, 16*(3), 42–51.

43. Elliott, A. J., & Church, M. A. (2003). A motivational analysis of defensive pessimism and self-handicapping. *Journal of Personality, 71*(3), 369–396.

Norem, J. K., & Cantor, N. (1986). Defensive pessimism: harnessing anxiety as motivation. *Journal of Personality and Social Psychology, 51*(6), 1208–1217.

44. Preskitt, D. (2017). Elie Wiesel notes the opposite of love is indifference. *BORGEN Magazine* (October 16).

45. Berscheid, E. (1966). Opinion change and communicator-communicatee similarity and dissimilarity. *Journal of Personality and Social Psychology, 4*(6), 670–680.

Mills, J., & Kimble, C. E. (1973). Opinion change as a function of perceived similarity of the communicator and subjectivity of the issue. *Bulletin of the Psychonomic Society, 2*(1), 35–36.

Simons, H. W., Berkowitz, N. N., & Moyer, R. J. (1970). Similarity, credibility, and attitude change: A review and a theory. *Psychological Bulletin, 73*(1), 1–16.

46. Sherif, M. (1953). The concept of reference groups in human relations. In M. Sherif & M. O. Wilson (Eds.), *Group relations at the crossroads*. Harper.

47. Stafford, J. E., & Cocanougher, A. B. (1977). Reference group theory. In *Selected aspects of consumer behavior: A summary from the perspective of different disciplines* (pp. 361–379). National Science Foundation, Directorate for Research Applications, Research Applied to National Needs.

48. We documented dozens of such positive sudden changes in Miller, W. R., & C'de Baca, J. (2001). *Quantum change: When epiphanies and sudden insights transform ordinary lives*. Guilford Press.

In a follow-up 10 years later, these transformations had not only persisted but grown. C'de Baca, J., & Wilbourne, P. (2004). Quantum change: Ten years later. *Journal of Clinical Psychology, 60*(5), 531–541.

Sudden transformations to the dark side are described in Nowinski, J. (2004). Evil by default: The origins of dark visions. *Journal of Clinical Psychology, 60*, 519–530.

49. Her firsthand accounts of these visions or "showings" and their aftereffects are recounted in her journal. Starr, M. (2013). *The showings of Julian of Norwich: A new translation*. Hampton Roads.

50. Kress, L., & Aue, T. (2017). The link between optimism bias and attention bias: A neurocognitive perspective. *Neuroscience and Biobehavioral Reviews, 80*, 688–702.

51. McNaughton-Cassill, M. E. (2001). The news media and psychological distress. *Anxiety, Stress and Coping, 14*(2), 193–211.

52. de Wit, L., van Straten, A., Lamers, F., Cuijpers, P., & Penninx, B. (2011). Are sedentary television watching and computer use behaviors associated with anxiety and depressive disorders? *Psychiatry Research, 186*(2–3), 239–243.

53. Bu, F., Steptoe, A., Mak, H. W., & Fancourt, D. (2021). Time use and mental health in UK adults during an 11-week COVID-19 lockdown: A panel analysis. *British Journal of Psychiatry, 219*(4), 551–556.

Al Omari, O., Al Sabei, S., Al Rawajfah, O., Abu Sharour, L., Aljohani, K., Alomari, K., . . . Al Zubidi, B. (2020). Prevalence and predictors of depression, anxiety, and stress among youth at the time of COVID-19: An online cross-sectional multicountry study. *Depression Research and Treatment* 2020.

54. Kelberer, L. J. A., Kraines, M. A., & Wells, T. T. (2018). Optimism, hope, and

attention for emotional stimuli. *Personality and Individual Differences, 124,* 84–90.

55. Aspinwall, L. G., & Brunhart, S. M. (1996). Distinguishing optimism from denial: Optimistic beliefs predict attention to health threats. *Personality and Social Psychology Bulletin, 22*(10), 993–1003.

    Radcliffe, N. M., & Klein, W. M. P. (2002). Dispositional, unrealistic, and comparative optimism: Differential relations with the knowledge and processing of risk information and beliefs about personal risk. *Personality and Social Psychology Bulletin, 28*(6), 836–846.

56. Schuckit, M. A. (1985). Ethanol-induced changes in body sway in men at high alcoholism risk. *Archives of General Psychiatry, 42*(4), 375–379.

57. Eng, M. Y., Schuckit, M. A., & Smith, T. L. (2005). The level of response to alcohol in daughters of alcoholics and controls. *Drug and Alcohol Dependence, 79*(1), 83–93.

    Schuckit, M. A., Tsuang, J. W., Anthenelli, R. M., Tipp, J. E., & Nurnberger Jr, J. (1996). Alcohol challenges in young men from alcoholic pedigrees and control families: A report from the COGA project. *Journal of Studies on Alcohol, 57*(4), 368–377.

58. *www.optimist.org/member/creed.cfm.*

59. Rafiq, F., Chishty, S. K., & Adil, M. (2022). Explanatory or dispositional optimism: Which trait predicts eco-friendly tourist behavior? *Sustainability, 14*(5).

    Yang, S., Markoczy, L., & Qi, M. (2007). Unrealistic optimism in consumer credit card adoption. *Journal of Economic Psychology, 28*(2), 170–185.

60. Anglin, A. H., McKenny, A. F., & Short, J. C. (2018). The impact of collective optimism on new venture creation and growth: A social contagion perspective. *Entrepreneurship Theory and Practice, 42*(3), 390–425.

    Catalano, R. A., Goldman-Mellor, S., Karasek, D. A., Gemmill, A., Casey, J. A., Elser, H., . . . & Hartig, T. (2020). Collective optimism and selection against male twins in utero. *Twin Research and Human Genetics, 23*(1), 45–50.

    Guèvremont, A., Boivin, C., Durif, F., & Graf, R. (2022). Positive behavioral change during the COVID-19 crisis: The role of optimism and collective resilience. *Journal of Consumer Behaviour, 21*(6), 1293–1306.

    Gürol, M., & Krimgil, S. (2010). Academic optimism. *Procedia-Social and Behavioral Sciences, 9,* 929–932.

61. Bennett, O. (2011). Cultures of optimism. *Cultural Sociology, 5*(2), 301–320.

    Watson, C. B., Chemers, M. M., & Preiser, N. (2001). Collective efficacy: A multilevel analysis. *Personality and Social Psychology Bulletin, 27*(8), 1057–1068.

62. Dunbar-Ortiz, R. (2014). *An indigenous people's history of the United States: ReVisioning history*. Beacon Press.

63. Kruger, J. (1999). Lake Wobegon be gone! The "below-average effect" and the egocentric nature of comparative ability judgments. *Journal of Personality and Social Psychology, 77*(2), 221–232.

64. Peterson, C. (2000). The future of optimism. *American Psychologist, 55*(1), 44–55.

CHAPTER 6. Trust

1. Erikson, E. H. (1950). *Childhood and society*. Norton.

2. Castonguay, L. G., & Hill, C. E. (Eds.). (2012). *Transformation in psychotherapy: Corrective experiences across cognitive behavioral, humanistic, and psychodynamic approaches*. American Psychological Association.

3. Miller, W. R., & Rollnick, S. (2023). *Motivational interviewing: Helping people change and grow*. Guilford Press.
   Price, D. D., Finniss, D. G., & Benedetti, F. (2008). A comprehensive review of the placebo effect: Recent advances and current thought. *Annual Review of Psychology, 59*(1), 565–590.

4. Yablonsky, L. (1965). *Synanon: The tunnel back*. Penguin Books.
   Janzen, R. (2001). *The rise and fall of Synanon*. Johns Hopkins University Press.

5. Mr. Roberts's method was adopted by Queen Elizabeth II as standard practice in England's royal stables.
   Roberts, M. (1997). *The man who listens to horses: The story of a real-life horse whisperer*. Random House.
   Roberts, M. (2013). *From my hands to yours: Lessons from a lifetime of training championship horses*. Monty & Pat Roberts.

6. Miller, W. R. (2000). Motivational interviewing: IV. Some parallels with horse whispering. *Behavioural and Cognitive Psychotherapy, 28*, 285–292.

7. The usual term is PTSD: Post-traumatic stress disorder. General Peter Chiarelli suggested instead that it should be called PTSI. A disorder is something that's wrong with you. An injury is something that happened to you.

8. Monty Roberts described and demonstrated his method in video recordings like *Join-up* and *Shy Boy*. Ailable from *https://montyroberts.com*.

9. Zinn, J. O. (2016). "In-between" and other reasonable ways to deal with risk and uncertainty: A review article. *Health, Risk & Society, 18*(7–8), 348–366.

10. Luke 2:8–20. (1989). *The Holy Bible: New Revised Standard Version*. Oxford University Press.

11. Growiec, K., & Growiec, J. (2014). Trusting only whom you know, knowing only whom you trust: The joint impact of social capital and trust on happiness in CEE countries. *Journal of Happiness Studies, 15*(5), 1015–1040.

    Tov, W., & Diener, E. (2008). The well-being of nations: Linking together trust, cooperation, and democracy. In B. A. Sullivan, M. Snyder, & J. L. Sullivan (Eds.), *Cooperation: The political psychology of effective human interaction* (pp. 323–342). Blackwell.

12. Dekker, P., & Broek, A. (2004). Civil society in longitudinal and comparative perspective: Voluntary associations, political involvement, social trust and happiness in a dozen countries. *Proceedings of the 6th International Conference of the International Society for Third-sector Research*. Ryerson University, Toronto, ON, Canada.

    Jasielska, D. (2020). The moderating role of kindness on the relation between trust and happiness. *Current Psychology, 39*(6), 2065–2073.

13. Neki, J. S. (1976). An examination of the cultural relativism of dependence as a dynamic of social and therapeutic relationships: I. Socio-developmental. *British Journal of Medical Psychology 49*(1), 1–10.

    Neki, J. (1976). An examination of the cultural relativism of dependence as a dynamic of social and therapeutic relationships: II. Therapeutic. *British Journal of Medical Psychology, 49*(1), 11–22.

14. Peterson, C., & Seligman, M. E. P. (Eds.). (2004). *Character strengths and virtues: A handbook and classification* (pp. 569–582). Oxford University Press.

    Smith, B. W. (2020). *Move from surviving to thriving: The positive psychology workbook for challenging times*. Independently published.

15. Cooperrider, D. L., & Whitney, D. (2005). *Appreciative inquiry: A positive revolution in change*. Berrett-Koehler.

    Bushe, G. R. (1999). Advances in appreciative inquiry as an organization development intervention. *Organization Development Journal, 17*(2), 61–68.

16. Goldberg, S. B., Babins-Wagner, R., Rousmaniere, T., Berzins, S., Hoyt, W. T., Whipple, J. L., . . . Wampold, B. E. (2016). Creating a climate for therapist improvement: A case study of an agency focused on outcomes and deliberate practice. *Psychotherapy, 53*(3), 367–375.

17. Shakespeare, W. *Julius Caesar,* Act 3, Scene 1.

18. Finley, J. (2023). *The healing path: A memoir and an invitation*. Orbis Books.

19. Mayer, R. C., Davis, J. H., & Schoorman, F. D. (1995). An integrative model of organizational trust. *Academy of Management Review, 20,* 709–734.

20. Fromm, E. (1968). *The revolution of hope: Toward a humanized technology.* Harper & Row. Quotation from p. 14.

21. Cohen, J. (1994). The earth is round (*p* < .05). *American Psychologist, 49,* 997–1003.
Cowles, M., & Davis, C. (1982). On the origins of the .05 level of statistical significance. *American Psychologist, 37,* 553–558.

22. Dunn, J. R., & Schweitzer, M. E. (2005). Feeling and believing: The influence of emotion on trust. *Journal of Personality and Social Psychology, 88*(5), 736–748.

23. Kraus, J., Scholz, D., Messner, E.-M., Messner, M., & Baumann, M. (2020). Scared to trust?–Predicting trust in highly automated driving by depressiveness, negative self-evaluations and state anxiety. *Frontiers in Psychology, 10,* 2917.

24. Lee, J. I., Dirks, K. T., & Campagna, R. L. (2023). At the heart of trust: Understanding the integral relationship between emotion and trust. *Group & Organization Management, 48*(2), 546–580.

25. Bar-Tal, D. (2001). Why does fear override hope in societies engulfed by intractable conflict, as it does in the Israeli society? *Political Psychology, 22*(3), 601–627.

26. Matthew 18:21–22. (1989). *The Holy Bible: New Revised Standard Version.* Oxford University Press. The answer has also been translated as *seventy times seven* or 490, further confounding our ability to keep score.

27. Chambers, J. R., & Windschitl, P. D. (2004). Biases in social comparative judgments: The role of nonmotivated factors in above-average and comparative-optimism effects. *Psychological Bulletin, 130*(5), 813–838.
Zell, E., Strickhouser, J. E., Sedikides, C., & Alicke, M. D. (2020). The better-than-average effect in comparative self-evaluation: A comprehensive review and meta-analysis. *Psychological Bulletin, 146*(2), 118–149.

28. Swenson, J. E., Schneller, G. R., & Henderson, J. A. (2014). The better-than-average effect and 1 Corinthians 13: A classroom exercise. *Christian Higher Education, 13*(2), 118–129.

29. Cross, K. P. (1977). Not can, but will college teaching be improved? *New Directions for Higher Education, 17,* 1–15.

30. Talsma, K., Schüz, B., & Norris, K. (2019). Miscalibration of self-efficacy and academic performance: Self-efficacy–self-fulfilling prophecy. *Learning and Individual Differences, 69,* 182–195.

31. Miller, W. R., & Moyers, T. B. (2021). *Effective psychotherapists: Clinical skills that improve client outcomes.* Guilford Press.
Tracey, T. J., Wampold, B. E., Lichtenberg, J. W., & Goodyear, R. K. (2014).

Expertise in psychotherapy: An elusive goal? *American Psychologist, 69*(3), 218–229.

32. Chow, D. L., Miller, S. D., Seidel, J. A., Kane, R. T., Thornton, J. A., & Andrews, W. P. (2015). The role of deliberate practice in the development of highly effective psychotherapists. *Psychotherapy, 52*(3), 337–345.

Rousmaniere, T., Goodyear, R. K., Miller, S. D., & Wampold, B. E. (2017). *The cycle of excellence: Using deliberate practice to improve supervision and training.* Wiley.

33. Miller, W. R., & Rollnick, S. (2023). *Motivational interviewing: Helping people change and grow.* Guilford Press.

34. Miller, W. R., & Mount, K. A. (2001). A small study of training in motivational interviewing: Does one workshop change clinician and client behavior? *Behavioural and Cognitive Psychotherapy, 29,* 457–471.

35. Dunning, D., Johnson, K., Ehrlinger, J., & Kruger, J. (2003). Why people fail to recognize their own incompetence. *Current Directions in Psychological Science, 12*(3), 83–87.

36. Miller, W. R., Yahne, C. E., Moyers, T. B., Martinez, J., & Pirritano, M. (2004). A randomized trial of methods to help clinicians learn motivational interviewing. *Journal of Consulting and Clinical Psychology, 72*(6), 1050–1062.

CHAPTER 7. Meaning And Purpose

1. *www.aruma.com.au/about-us/blog/christopher-reeve-the-life-of-the-man-of-steel. Accessed on 8/2/2023*

2. Park, C. L., & Folkman, S. (1997). Meaning in the context of stress and coping. *Review of General Psychology, 1*(2), 115–144.

3. "If a man's ego has been stabilized, resulting in a sure grounding of his sense of personal worth and dignity . . . he can think of himself with some measure of detachment from the shackles of his immediate world. . . . The fact that he is denied opportunity will not necessarily deter him." Quoted in Thurman, H. (1976). *Jesus and the disinherited*, p. 43. Beacon Press.

4. Quoted from "I've Been to the Mountaintop" by Dr. Martin Luther King Jr. American Federation of State, County and Municipal Employees (AFSCME). *www.afscme.org/about/history/mlk/mountaintop*

5. Jeremiah, D. (2021). *Hope: Living fearlessly in a scary world.* Tyndale.

Pinsent, A. (2020). Hope as a virtue in the Middle Ages. In S. C. van den Heuvel (Ed.), *Historical and multidisciplinary perspectives on hope* (pp. 47–60). Springer Open.

6. Alcoholics Anonymous World Services. (2001). *Alcoholics Anonymous: The story of how many thousands of men and women have recovered from alcoholism* (4th ed.). Author.

   Kurtz, E. (1991). *Not-God: A history of Alcoholics Anonymous* (Expanded ed.). Hazelden.

7. Alaszewski, A., & Wilkinson, I. (2015). The paradox of hope for working age adults recovering from stroke. *Health (London), 19*(2), 172–187.

8. Wayland, S., Maple, M., McKay, K., & Glassock, G. (2016). Holding on to hope: A review of the literature exploring missing persons, hope and ambiguous loss. *Death Studies, 40*(1), 54–60.

9. Frankl, V. E. (1969). *The will to meaning.* World.

   Frankl, V. E. (2006). *Man's search for meaning.* Beacon Press.

   Redsand, A. S. (2006). *Viktor Frankl: A life worth living.* Clarion Books.

10. Kylmä, J., & Juvakka, T. (2007). Hope in parents of adolescents with cancer—Factors endangering and engendering parental hope. *European Journal of Oncology Nursing, 11*(3), 262–271.

11. That there is no inherent meaning in life and we are free to make our own is a classic philosophic view in existentialism. Sartre, J. P. (2007). *Existentialism is a humanism.* Yale University Press.

12. Miller, W. R. (2004). The phenomenon of quantum change. *Journal of Clinical Psychology, 60*(5), 453–460.

    Miller, W. R., & C'de Baca, J. (2001). *Quantum change: When epiphanies and sudden insights transform ordinary lives.* Guilford Press.

13. C'de Baca, J., & Wilbourne, P. (2004). Quantum change: Ten years later. *Journal of Clinical Psychology, 60*, 531–541.

14. Greyson, B. (2021). *After: A doctor explores what near-death experiences reveal about life and beyond.* St. Martin's Essentials.

15. Pargament, K. I., & Exline, J. J. (2022). *Working with spiritual struggles in psychotherapy: From research to practice.* Guilford Press.

16. Wiking, M. (2017). *The little book of hygge: Danish secrets to happy living.* William Morrow.

17. Webb, D. (2007). Modes of hoping. *History of the Human Sciences, 20*(3), 65–83.

18. These are the concluding words of Pierre Teilhard de Chardin's *How I believe* (1969). William Collins & Sons.

19. Rohr, R. (2001). *Hope against darkness: The transforming vision of Saint Francis in an age of anxiety.* St. Anthony Messenger Press.

20. Cohen, R., Bavishi, C., & Rozanski, A. (2016). Purpose in life and its relationship to all-cause mortality and cardiovascular events: A meta-analysis. *Psychosomatic Medicine, 78*(2), 122–133.

Hill, P. L., & Turiano, N. A. (2014). Purpose in life as a predictor of mortality across adulthood. *Psychological Science, 25*(7), 1482–1486.

McKnight, P. E., & Kashdan, T. B. (2009). Purpose in life as a system that creates and sustains health and well-being: An integrative, testable theory. *Review of General Psychology, 13*(3), 242–251.

Pfund, G. N., & Hill, P. L. (2018). The multifaceted benefits of purpose in life. *International Forum for Logotherapy, 41*(1), 27–37.

Reker, G. T., Peacock, E. J., & Wong, P. T. (1987). Meaning and purpose in life and well-being: A life-span perspective. *Journal of Gerontology, 42*(1), 44–49.

21. Feldman, D. B., & Snyder, C. R. (2005). Hope and the meaningful life: Theoretical and empirical associations between goal-directed thinking and life meaning. *Journal of Social and Clinical Psychology, 24*(3), 401–421.

Gan, L. L., Gong, S., & Kissane, D. W. (2022). Mental state of demoralisation across diverse clinical settings: A systematic review, meta-analysis and proposal for its use as a "specifier" in mental illness. *Australian & New Zealand Journal of Psychiatry, 56*(9), 1104–1129.

22. Miller, W. R., & Harris, R. J. (2000). A simple scale of Gorski's warning signs for relapse. *Journal of Studies on Alcohol, 61,* 759–765.

23. Irving, J., Davis, S., & Collier, A. (2017). Aging with purpose: Systematic search and review of literature pertaining to older adults and purpose. *International Journal of Aging and Human Development, 85*(4), 403–437.

24. Sutin, A. R., Aschwanden, D., Luchetti, M., Stephan, Y., & Terracciano, A. (2021). Sense of purpose in life is associated with lower risk of incident dementia: A meta-analysis. *Journal of Alzheimer's Disease, 83*(1), 249–258.

Sutin, A. R., Aschwanden, D., Luchetti, M., Stephan, Y., & Terracciano, A. (2021). Sense of purpose in life is associated with lower risk of incident dementia: A meta-analysis. *Journal of Alzheimer's Disease, 83*(1), 249–258.

25. Kim, E. S., Strecher, V. J., & Ryff, C. D. (2014). Purpose in life and use of preventive health care services. *Proceedings of the National Academy of Sciences, 111*(46), 16331–16336.

26. Pinquart, M. (2002). Creating and maintaining purpose in life in old age: A meta-analysis. *Ageing International, 27*(2), 90–114.

27. Griggs, S., & Walker, R. K. (2016). The role of hope for adolescents with a chronic illness: An integrative review. *Journal of Pediatric Nursing, 31*(4), 404–421.

28. Scales, R., Lueker, R. D., Atterbom, H. A., Handmaker, N. S., & Jackson, K. A. (1997). Impact of motivational interviewing and skills-based counseling on outcomes in cardiac rehabilitation. *Journal of Cardiopulmonary Rehabilitation, 17.*

29. Brueggemann, W. (2001). *The prophetic imagination* (2nd ed.). Fortress Press.

30. Jeremiah 29:5–7. (1989). *The Holy Bible: New Revised Standard Version.* Oxford University Press.

31. Boukala, S., & Dimitrakopoulou, D. (2017). The politics of fear vs. the politics of hope: Analysing the 2015 Greek election and referendum campaigns. *Critical Discourse, 14*(1), 39–55.

    Miller, W. R. (2022). *On second thought: How ambivalence shapes your life.* Guilford Press.

CHAPTER 8. Perseverance

1. Elliot, D. (2020). Hope in theology. In S. C. van den Heuvel (Ed.), *Historical and multidisciplinary perspectives on hope* (pp. 117–136). Springer Open.

2. Rollnick, S., Miller, W. R., & Butler, C. C. (2023). *Motivational interviewing in health care* (2nd ed.). Guilford Press.

3. Milona, M. (2020). Philosophy of hope. In S. C. van den Heuvel (Ed.), *Historical and multidisciplinary perspectives on hope* (pp. 99–116). Springer Open.

    In philosophy, belief in one's ability to effect change is called *agency*. In psychology, the popular term is *self-efficacy*.

    Bandura, A. (1982). Self-efficacy mechanism in human agency. *American Psychologist, 37,* 122–147.

    Bandura, A. (1997). *Self-efficacy: The exercise of control.* Freeman.

4. Peterson, C., Maier, S. F., & Seligman, M. E. P. (1995). *Learned helplessness: A theory for the age of personal control.* Oxford University Press.

    Maier, S. F., & Seligman, M. E. (2016). Learned helplessness at fifty: Insights from neuroscience. *Psychological Review, 123*(4), 349–367.

5. Maier, S. F. (1984). Learned helplessness and animal models of depression. *Progress in Neuro-Psychopharmacology and Biological Psychiatry, 8*(3), 435–446.

    Miller, W. R., & Seligman, M. E. (1975). Depression and learned helplessness in man. *Journal of Abnormal Psychology, 84*(3), 228–238.

6. Hibbard, J. H., Mahoney, E. R., Stock, R., & Tusler, M. (2007). Do increases in patient activation result in improved self-management behaviors? *Health Services Research, 42*(4), 1443–1463.

Moore, M., Wolever, R., Hibbard, J., & Lawson, K. (2012). *Three pillars of health coaching: Patient activation, motivational interviewing and positive psychology.* Healthcare Intelligence Network.

7. Lewinsohn, P. M., Muñoz, R. F., Youngren, M. A., & Zeiss, A. M. (1992). *Control your depression* (rev. ed.). Fireside.

Dimidjian, S., Barrera, M., Jr., Martell, C., Muñoz, R. F., & Lewinsohn, P. M. (2011). The origins and current status of behavioral activation treatments for depression. *Annual Review of Clinical Psychology, 7,* 1–38.

8. Daugherty, M. D. (2003). *A randomized trial of motivational interviewing with college students for academic success.* PhD dissertation, University of New Mexico, Albuquerque.

9. Brent, D. A., Brunwasser, S. M., Hollon, S. D., Weersing, V. R., Clarke, G. N., Dickerson, J. F., . . . & Lynch, F. L. (2015). Effect of a cognitive-behavioral prevention program on depression 6 years after implementation among at-risk adolescents: A randomized clinical trial. *JAMA Psychiatry, 72*(11), 1110–1118.

Pozza, A., & Dèttore, D. (2020). Modular cognitive-behavioral therapy for affective symptoms in young individuals at ultra-high risk of first episode of psychosis: Randomized controlled trial. *Journal of Clinical Psychology, 76*(3), 392–405.

Sockol, L. E. (2015). A systematic review of the efficacy of cognitive behavioral therapy for treating and preventing perinatal depression. *Journal of Affective Disorders, 177,* 7–21.

10. Romans 5:4. (1989). *The Holy Bible: New Revised Standard Version.* Oxford University Press.

11. Yotsidi, V., Pagoulatou, A., Kyriazos, T., & Stalikas, A. (2018). The role of hope in academic and work environments: An integrative literature review. *Psychology, 9*(3), 385–402.

12. Reichard, R. J., Avey, J. B., Lopez, S., & Dollwet, M. (2013). Having the will and finding the way: A review and meta-analysis of hope at work. *Journal of Positive Psychology, 8*(4), 292–304.

13. Kortte, K. B., Stevenson, J. E., Hosey, M. M., Castillo, R., & Wegener, S. T. (2012). Hope predicts positive functional role outcomes in acute rehabilitation populations. *Rehabilitation Psychology, 57*(3), 248–255.

14. Gollwitzer, P. M. (1999). Implementation intentions: Strong effects of simple plans. *American Psychologist, 54*(7), 493–503.

Gollwitzer, P. M., Wieber, F., Myers, A. L., & McCrea, S. M. (2010). How to maximize implementation intention effects. In C. R. Agnew, D. E. Carlston, W. G. Graziano, & J. R. Kelly (Eds.), *Then a miracle occurs: Focusing on behavior in social psychological theory and research* (pp. 137–161). Oxford University Press.

15. Gillham, J. E., Shatté, A. J., Reivich, K. J., & Seligman, M. E. (2001). Optimism, pessimism, and explanatory style. In E. C. Chang (Ed.), *Optimism and pessimism: Implications for theory, research, and practice* (pp. 53–75). American Psychological Association.

    Zimmerman, M. A. (1990). Toward a theory of learned hopefulness: A structural model analysis of participation and empowerment. *Journal of Research in Personality, 24*(1), 71–86.

16. Lybbert, T. J., & Wydick, B. (2018). Poverty, aspirations, and the economics of hope. *Economic Development and Cultural Change, 66*(4), 709–753.

17. Biographical information from the Wikipedia entry on J. K. Rowling, downloaded on August 14, 2023.

18. Masten, A. S. (2014). Global perspectives on resilience in children and youth. *Child Development, 85*(1), 6–20.

    Lybbert, T. J., & Wydick, B. (2018). Poverty, aspirations, and the economics of hope. *Economic Development and Cultural Change, 66*(4), 709–753.

19. Armor, D. A., & Taylor, S. E. (1998). Situated optimism: Specific outcome expectancies and self-regulation. In M. P. Zanna (Ed.), *Advances in Experimental Social Psychology* (Vol. 30, pp. 309–379). Academic Press.

20. Luthans, F., Avey, J. B., Avolio, B. J., & Peterson, S. J. (2010). The development and resulting performance impact of positive psychological capital. *Human Resource Development Quarterly, 21*(1), 41–67.

21. Martin Luther King Jr., *Letter from a Birmingham Jail,* April 16, 1963.

22. Armor, D. A., & Taylor, S. E. (1998). Situated optimism: Specific outcome expectancies and self-regulation. In M. P. Zanna (Ed.), *Advances in Experimental Social Psychology* (vol. 30, pp. 309–379). Academic Press.

23. McCullough, D. (1977). *The path between the seas: The creation of the Panama Canal 1870–1914.* Simon & Schuster.

24. Singer/songwriter Don Eaton captured this moment in his lyric: "I was a witness to the sacrament, child with a bucket in his hand. He brought the holy water from the sea to the giants dying in the sand. It was the ancient ceremony. He did not need to understand." I first told this story in *Living As If: How Positive Faith Can Change Your Life* (Wipf & Stock, reprinted 2020).

CHAPTER 9. Hope Beyond Hope

1. Havel, V. (1990). *Letters to Olga* (Paul Wilson, Trans.). Faber & Faber. Martin Luther King Jr. similarly wrote, in a letter from the Birmingham jail, "I have no despair about the future." John Lewis reported that Dr. King told his followers from time to time, "If you don't have hope, you're already dead. You're not really here." Quoted in Dear. J. (2022). Nonviolence is Christian love in action: A conversation with John Lewis. *Oneing: An Alternative Orthodoxy, 10*(2), 39–46. Center for Action and Contemplation.

2. A first-century use of the phrase "hoping against hope" describes the hope of the Hebrew patriarch Abraham, as a childless old man, to have many descendants (Romans 4:18).

3. As Barack Obama famously said, "Hope is that thing inside us that insists, despite all the evidence to the contrary, that something better awaits us if we have the courage to reach for it and to work for it and to fight for it." From his Iowa caucus speech quoted in the *New York Times*, January 3, 2008.

4. Tillich, P. (1965). The right to hope. *University of Chicago Magazine, 58*(2), 16–21. This was apparently Tillich's last sermon.

5. Zinn, J. O. (2016). "In-between" and other reasonable ways to deal with risk and uncertainty: A review article. *Health, Risk and Society, 18*(7–8), 348–366.

6. Marcel, G. (1951). *Homo viator: Introduction to a metaphysic of hope.* Harper & Row.

7. Robertson, D. (1975). *Sea survival: A manual.* Praeger.

8. Buber, M. (1971). *I and thou.* Free Press.
   Miller, W. R. (2017). *Lovingkindness: Realizing and practicing your true self.* Wipf & Stock.
   Salzberg, S. (1995). *Lovingkindness: The revolutionary art of happiness.* Shambhala.
   The Dalai Lama, & Vreeland, N. (2001). *An open heart: Practicing compassion in everyday life.* Little, Brown.

9. Frank, A. *The diary of a young girl,* entry from Saturday, July 15, 1944, p. 358.

10. Venter, S. (Ed.). (2018). *The prison letters of Nelson Mandela.* Liveright.

11. This ultimate hope in the movement of history toward a meaningful and benevolent omega point is found throughout the writings of Pierre Teilhard de Chardin, including *The future of man* (1964), *Toward the future* (1975), and *The phenomenon of man* (2008).

12. Macy, J., & Johnstone, C. (2022). *Active hope: How to face the mess we're in with unexpected resilience & creative power* (rev. ed.). New World Library.

13. Miller, W. R., & Rollnick, S. (2023). *Motivational interviewing: Helping people change and grow* (4th ed.). Guilford Press.

14. Miller, W. R. (1985). *Living as if: How positive faith can change your life.* Westminster Press. (Republished in 2020 by Wipf & Stock.)

    Miller, W. R., & Jackson, K. A. (1995). *Practical psychology for pastors: Toward more effective counseling.* (2nd ed.). Prentice-Hall. (Republished in 2010 by Wipf & Stock.)

    Miller, W. R. (Ed.). (1999). *Integrating spirituality into treatment: Resources for practitioners.* American Psychological Association.

    Miller, W. R., & Thoresen, C. E. (2003). Spirituality, religion, and health: An emerging research field. *American Psychologist, 58,* 24–35.

    Miller, W. R., & Delaney, H. D. (Eds.) (2005). *Judeo-Christian perspectives on psychology: Human nature, motivation, and change.* American Psychological Association.

15. Miller, W. R., & C'de Baca, J. (2001). *Quantum change: When epiphanies and sudden insights transform ordinary lives.* Guilford Press.

16. Enduring life transformations do sometimes occur when people pray in desperate circumstances, perhaps for the first time in their lives. Such a story is that of Bill Wilson, who, on the brink of death from chronic alcoholism, had a dramatic "white light" experience and not only stopped drinking, but permanently lost his desire for alcohol. He went on to become the cofounder of Alcoholics Anonymous.

17. Bidney, M. (2004). Epiphany in autobiography: The quantum changes of Dostoevsky and Tolstoy. *Journal of Clinical Psychology, 60,* 471–480.

18. Mackesy, C. (2019). *The boy, the mole, the fox and the horse.* Harper One.

19. Adapted with permission from W. R. Miller (2017). *Lovingkindness: Realizing and practicing your true self.* Cascade Books (Wipf & Stock).

20. LaMotte, D. (2014). *Worldchanging 101: Challenging the myth of powerlessness.* Dryad.

21. Braithwaite, V. (2004). Collective hope. *Annals of the American Academy of Political and Social Science, 592,* 6–15.

    Peterson, C. (2000). The future of optimism. *American Psychologist, 55*(1), 44–55.

22. As recounted to his friend, John Dear, in Dear, J. (2013). *The nonviolent life.*

Pace e Bene Press. His own account is Zinn, H. (2015), *A people's history of the United States,* HarperCollins.

23. Isaiah 2:4. (1989). *The Holy Bible: New Revised Standard Version.* Oxford University Press.

24. An "anti-determinist" perspective affirms that change is still possible. Webb, D. (2007). Modes of hoping. *History of the Human Sciences, 20*(3), 65–83.

25. Dear, J. (2013). *The nonviolent life.* Pace e Bene Press.

26. Benson, H., & Kipper, M. Z. (2000). *The relaxation response.* HarperCollins.
    Bourgeault, C. (2004). *Centering prayer and inner awakening.* Cowley.
    Kabat-Zinn, J. (1994). *Wherever you go, there you are: Mindfulness meditation in everyday life.* Hachette.
    Nhat Hanh, T. (2015). *The miracle of mindfulness: An introduction to the practice of meditation* (Mobi Ho, Trans.). Beacon Press.

27. Elliott, R., Bohart, A. C., Watson, J. C., & Murphy, D. (2018). Therapist empathy and client outcome: An updated meta-analysis. *Psychotherapy, 55*(4), 399–410.
    Miller, W. R. (2018). *Listening well: The art of empathic understanding.* Wipf & Stock.
    Rogers, C. R. (1980). Empathic: An unappreciated way of being. In C. R. Rogers (Ed.), *A way of being* (pp. 137–163). Houghton Mifflin.

28. Sánchez-Rojo, A. (2022). Waiting before hoping: An educational approach to the experience of waiting. *Educational Philosophy and Theory, 54*(1), 71–80.

CHAPTER 10. Choosing Hope

1. Delio, I. (2013). *The unbearable wholeness of being: God, evolution, and the power of love.* Orbis Books.

2. Frank, A. *The diary of a young girl,* entry from June 6,1944, p. 336.

3. John 21:1–14. (1989). *The Holy Bible: New Revised Standard Version.* Oxford University Press.

4. The rest of our story is told in W. R Miller & L. K. Homer (2016), *Portals: Two lives intertwined by adoption.* Wipf & Stock.

5. Miller, W. R., & C'de Baca, J. (1994). Quantum change: Toward a psychology of transformation. In T. Heatherton & J. Weinberger (Eds.), *Can personality change?* (pp. 253–280). American Psychological Association.
   Miller, W. R., & C'de Baca, J. (2001). *Quantum change: When epiphanies and sudden insights transform ordinary lives.* Guilford Press.

6. Frankl, V. E. (2006). *Man's search for meaning.* Beacon Press.

7. Greyson, B. (2021). *After: A doctor explores what near-death experiences reveal about life and beyond.* St. Martin's Essentials.

   Miller, W. R., & C'de Baca, J. (2001). *Quantum change: When epiphanies and sudden insights transform ordinary lives.* Guilford Press.

8. Kirschenbaum, H. (2013). *Values clarification: Practical strategies for individual and group settings.* Oxford University Press.

   Rokeach, M. (1973). *The nature of human values.* Free Press.

   Simon, S. B., Howe, L. W., & Kirschenbaum, H. (1995). *Values clarification: A practical, action-directed workbook.* Warner Books.

9. Tillich, P. (1965). The right to hope. *University of Chicago Magazine, 58*(2), 16–21.

10. Dickinson, J. K. (2013). *People with diabetes can eat anything: It's all about balance.* Media 117.

11. Miller, W. R., & Hester, R. K. (1986). Inpatient alcoholism treatment: Who benefits? *American Psychologist, 41,* 794–805.

12. Marlatt, G. A., & Donovan, D. M. (Eds.). (2005). *Relapse prevention: Maintenance strategies in the treatment of addictive behaviors* (2nd ed.). Guilford Press.

13. I have argued that we should retire the idea of "relapse" in addiction treatment. It's merely substance use, the primary symptom in substance use disorders, and imperfection is the norm in human nature. Relabeling any use as a failure or a relapse adds arbitrary moral and emotional baggage.

    Miller, W. R. (1996). What is a relapse? Fifty ways to leave the wagon. *Addiction, 91* (Suppl.), S15–S27.

    Miller, W. R. (2015). Retire the concept of "relapse." *Substance Use and Misuse, 50*(8–9), 976–977.

    Miller, W. R., Forcehimes, A. A., & Zweben, A. (2019). *Treating addiction: A guide for professionals* (2nd ed.). Guilford Press.

14. Miller, W. R., Walters, S. T., & Bennett, M. E. (2001). How effective is alcoholism treatment in the United States? *Journal of Studies on Alcohol, 62,* 211–220.

15. Hastie, R., & Dawes, R. M. (2009). *Rational choice in an uncertain world: The psychology of judgment and decision making* (2nd ed.). Sage.

    Kahneman, D. (2011). *Thinking, fast and slow.* Farrar, Straus and Giroux.

    Tversky, A., & Kahneman, D. (1974). Judgment under uncertainty: Heuristics and biases. *Science, 185*(4157), 1124–1131.

16. Miller, W. R. (1976). Alcoholism scales and objective assessment methods: A review. *Psychological Bulletin, 83,* 649–674.

17. *The Man of La Mancha* was a 1960s play written by Dale Wasserman that
     became a highly popular Broadway musical by Joe Darion and Mitch Leigh.
     Half a century later its message of hope continues in ongoing performances.

18. Beck, J. S., & Beck, A. T. (2011). *Cognitive behavior therapy: Basics and beyond*
     (2nd ed.). Guilford Press.

     Burns, D. D. (1999). *Feeling good: The clinically proven drug-free treatment for
     depression* (rev. ed.). William Morrow.

     Leahy, R. L. (2017). *Cognitive therapy techniques: A practitioner's guide* (2nd
     ed.). Guilford Press.

     Lewinsohn, P. M., Muñoz, R. F., Youngren, M. A., & Zeiss, A. M. (1992). *Control
     your depression* (rev. ed.). Fireside.

19. Fetzer Institute. (1999). *Multidimensional measurement of religiousness/spirituality
     for use in health research*. Author.

20. Emmons, R. A., & McCullough, R. W. (2004). *The psychology of gratitude*.
     Oxford University Press.

     Sacks, O. (2015). *Gratitude*. Knopf.

21. From W. R. Miller & J. C'de Baca (2001). *Quantum change: When epiphanies
     and sudden insights transform ordinary lives*. Guilford Press. Quotation from
     p. 44.

22. Hupkens, S., Machielse, A., Goumans, M., & Derkx, P. (2018). Meaning in life
     of older persons: An integrative literature review. *Nursing Ethics, 25*(8), 973–
     991.

     Li, J.-B., Wang, Y.-S., Dou, K., & Shang, Y.-F. (2022). On the development of
     meaning in life among college freshmen: Social relationship antecedents and
     adjustment consequences. *Journal of Happiness Studies*, 1–27.

     O'Donnell, M. B., Bentele, C. N., Grossman, H. B., Le, Y., Jang, H., & Steger,
     M. F. (2014). You, me, and meaning: An integrative review of connections
     between relationships and meaning in life. *Journal of Psychology in Africa,
     24*(1), 44–50.

23. Baines, S., Saxby, P., & Ehlert, K. (1987). Reality orientation and reminiscence
     therapy: A controlled cross-over study of elderly confused people. *British Journal
     of Psychiatry, 151*(2), 222–231.

     Bhar, S. S. (2014). Reminiscence therapy: A review. In N. A. Pachana & K.
     Laidlaw (Eds.), *Oxford handbook of clinical geropsychology* (pp. 675–690).
     Oxford University Press.

     Chin, A. M. (2007). Clinical effects of reminiscence therapy in older adults: A
     meta-analysis of controlled trials. *Hong Kong Journal of Occupational Therapy,
     17*(1), 10–22.

Fujiwara, E., Otsuka, K., Sakai, A., Hoshi, K., Sekiai, S., Kamisaki, M., . . . & Chida, F. (2012). Usefulness of reminiscence therapy for community mental health. *Psychiatry and Clinical Neurosciences, 66*(1), 74–79.

24. Czyżowska, N., & Gurba, E. (2022). Enhancing meaning in life and psychological well-being among a European cohort of young adults via a gratitude intervention. *Frontiers in Psychology, 12.*

25. For example, there is a good variety of effective methods available for treating problems with alcohol and other drugs.

    Miller, W. R., Forcehimes, A. A., & Zweben, A. (2019). *Treating addiction: A guide for professionals* (2nd ed.). Guilford Press.

26. Lewis, C. S. (1960). *The four loves.* Harcourt Brace.

    Psaris, J., & Lyons, M. S. (2000). *Undefended love.* New Harbinger.

    Rohr, R. (2014). *Eager to love: The alternative way of Francis of Assisi.* Franciscan Media.

27. Folkman, S. (2010). Stress, coping, and hope. *Psycho-Oncology, 19*(9), 901–908.

28. Herth, K. A. (2001). Development and implementation of a hope intervention program. *Oncology Nursing Forum, 28*(6), 1009–1017.

    Lomranz, J., & Benyamini, Y. (2016). The ability to live with incongruence: Aintegration—The concept and its operationalization. *Journal of Adult Development, 23*(2), 79–92.

    Zinn, J. O. (2016). "In-between" and other reasonable ways to deal with risk and uncertainty: A review article. *Health, Risk & Society, 18*(7–8), 348–366.

29. Herth, K. A., & Cutcliffe, J. R. (2002). The concept of hope in nursing 3: Hope and palliative care nursing. *British Journal of Nursing, 11*(14), 977–982.

    Kirkpatrick, H., Landeen, J., Byrne, C., Woodside, H., Pawlick, J., & Bernardo, A. (1995). Hope and schizophrenia: Clinicians identify hope-instilling strategies. *Journal of Psychosocial Nursing and Mental Health Services, 33*(6), 15–41.

30. Esteves, M., Scoloveno, R. L., Mahat, G., Yarcheski, A., & Scoloveno, M. A. (2013). An integrative review of adolescent hope. *Journal of Pediatric Nursing, 28*(2), 105–113.

    Johnson, J. G., Alloy, L. B., Panzarella, C., Metalsky, G. I., Rabkin, J. G., Williams, J. B., & Abramson, L. Y. (2001). Hopelessness as a mediator of the association between social support and depressive symptoms: Findings of a study of men with HIV. *Journal of Consulting and Clinical Psychology, 69*(6), 1056–1060.

    Kirkpatrick, H., Landeen, J., Woodside, H., & Byrne, C. (2001). How people with schizophrenia build their hope. *Journal of Psychosocial Nursing and Mental Health Services 39*(1), 46–55.

31. Edey, W., & Jevne, R. F. (2003). Hope, illness, and counselling practice: Making hope visible. *Canadian Journal of Counselling, 37*(1), 44–51.

Larsen, D., Edey, W., & Lemay, L. (2007). Understanding the role of hope in counselling: Exploring the intentional uses of hope. *Counselling Psychology Quarterly, 20*(4), 401–416.

32. Braithwaite, V. (2004). Collective hope. *Annals of the American Academy of Political and Social Science, 592*, 6–15.

Schrank, B., Bird, V., Rudnick, A., & Slade, M. (2012). Determinants, self-management strategies and interventions for hope in people with mental disorders: Systematic search and narrative review. *Social Science and Medicine, 74*(4), 554–564.

Index

About the Author

William R. Miller, PhD, is Emeritus Distinguished Professor of Psychology and Psychiatry at the University of New Mexico. Fundamentally interested in the psychology of change, he cofounded the counseling method of Motivational Interviewing. He is a recipient of two career achievement awards from the American Psychological Association, the international Jellinek Memorial Award, and an Innovators Award from the Robert Wood Johnson Foundation, among many other honors.